Abba Goold Woolson

Dress-Reform

A series of lectures delivered in Boston, on dress as it affects the health of women

Abba Goold Woolson

Dress-Reform
A series of lectures delivered in Boston, on dress as it affects the health of women

ISBN/EAN: 9783337295721

Printed in Europe, USA, Canada, Australia, Japan

Cover: Foto ©Suzi / pixelio.de

More available books at **www.hansebooks.com**

DRESS-REFORM.

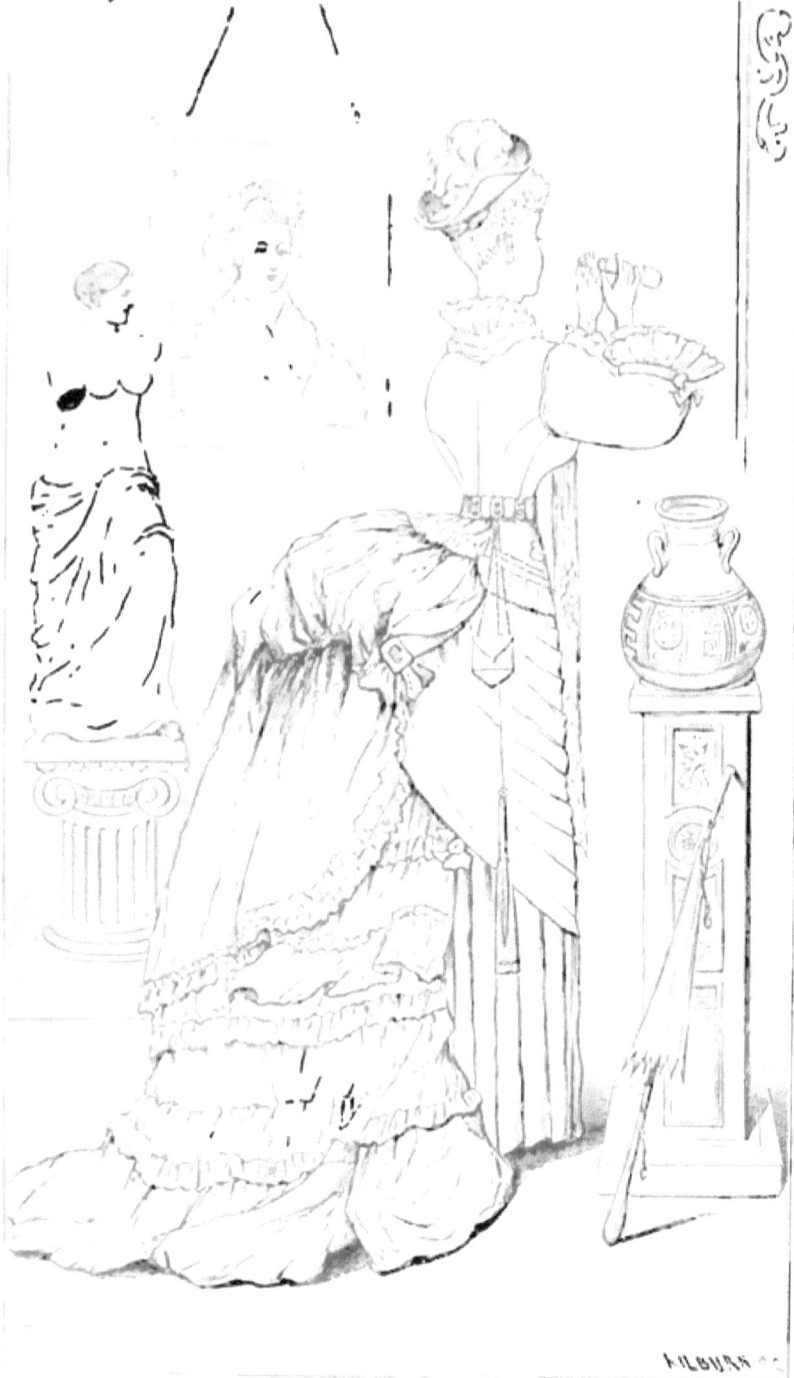

A SERIES OF LECTURES DELIVERED IN BOSTON,

ON DRESS AS IT AFFECTS THE HEALTH OF WOMEN.

EDITED BY
ABBA GOOLD WOOLSON.

With Illustrations.

BOSTON:
ROBERTS BROTHERS.
1874.

Entered according to Act of Congress, in the year 1874, by
ABBA GOOLD WOOLSON,
In the Office of the Librarian of Congress, at Washington.

Cambridge:
Press of John Wilson & Son.

INTRODUCTION.

The following Lectures were delivered in Boston during the spring of the present year; and their purpose was to arouse women to a knowledge of physical laws, to show them how their dress defies these laws, and what different garments they should adopt. All, save the last, were written by female physicians of recognized ability and position; and the testimony thus given concerning the injuries inflicted by dress was felt to be authoritative and convincing. The lectures excited much attention at their first presentation; and, soon after, they were repeated by request in several adjoining cities. In compliance with the wishes of many hearers, and from a desire to extend the good work which they have already accomplished, they are now offered to the public in permanent form.

It is believed that their force and value will be enhanced by a statement of the circumstances which led to their preparation.

A little over a year ago, it became the duty

of a committee of ladies, associated together, to take cognizance of the wide-spread and increasing dissatisfaction then existing in regard to woman's dress, to inquire into the many charges brought against it, and to determine what steps, if any, could be taken towards making it more healthful, artistic, and serviceable. With no preconceived theories to establish, these ladies set to work in good faith to ascertain precisely what was wrong, how to cure it, and how to render these cures acceptable and widely known. They consulted the experienced, fair-minded women about them, corresponded with many in other cities, and made a patient study of the hygienic and æsthetic principles to which a proper dress must conform. The result of these inquiries was to convince them that the whole structure and the essential features of our present apparel are undeniably opposed to the plainest requirements of health, beauty, and convenience, and that any remedies, to be thorough, must concern themselves not merely with the external costume, but with every garment worn beneath it.

It seemed vital to the physical well-being of the whole nation that such remedies, when devised, should be generally and permanently adopted. And yet it was also evident that any reform in woman's dress, which should produce a marked and sudden alteration in her appearance, would find favor with but a few; and that these few, however heroic, must ultimately yield to the prejudices of the many. Thus the wisest efforts would result in defeat, unless due deference were paid to the force of custom and to the conventional standards by which every innovation must be judged.

It was accordingly deemed best to render the improvements that should be recommended, however thorough they might be, as unnoticeable to ordinary observers as it was possible to make them, without too great a sacrifice of health, comfort, and beauty to the fashions of the time. A striking change in the appearance could only be produced by some sudden change in the external costume; and, tried by physiological principles, that appeared by no means the most objectionable portion of the attire. Indeed, under intelligent guidance, it would admit of such modifications and selections as would eliminate its worst features, and accommodate it to a wholly novel hygienic suit worn beneath it. And a complete revolution in the structure and the adjustment of the ordinary under-dress was by far the most important thing to be gained. If that could be effected, the outward covering would in time take care of itself.

This view did not imply that a radical change in the entire dress was not in itself desirable, but that, whether desirable or not, it could not be imposed at the present time. A new costume, to be of lasting benefit, must appear in response to a general call, and to meet an enlightened and permanent desire. Any endeavor to introduce it to-day would only invite another defeat, to dishearten reformers in the future.

The wisdom of these conclusions had been demonstrated by experience. All previous attempts at dress-reform had been failures, because they sought to accomplish an immediate result by ill-considered and inadequate means. It was supposed that from bad clothes to good was but a step, and that the only preliminaries necessary were to devise the best possible apparel, and to invite everybody to adopt it. The most noticeable of these failures was the Bloomer costume; for, of all attempted revolutions in dress, it sought to bring about the most radical change in the appearance, and it came the nearest to effecting this end. Its originators, who were themselves intelligent and brave, proceeded on the assumption that great numbers of women throughout the country were not only dissatisfied with the old attire and longing for a better, but that they would at once adopt a better as soon as it should appear, however odd it might look, and from whatever source it should spring. Others were to follow their example, not from any deliberate and reasoning preference for the new over the old, but because the new should become the mode. When all had worn it and experienced its blessings, they would refuse to abandon it, and thus its reign would be made secure.

The result proved how mistaken were these assumptions. It was, indeed, true that many had grown restless under the burdens and restrictions of their dress. Of these, the more desperate seized the remedy offered, and defied consequences; but a greater number, who coveted the ease and freedom it promised, lacked the courage to adopt it, and waited till it should establish itself in general favor. A few, regardless of higher claims, were attracted by its novelty, and hastened to lead a new style. But to the majority of thoughtless women it remained an object of indifference or of ridicule. With evils and their remedies they had little to do.

For them, nothing could be right which was not fashionable; and nothing could be fashionable which had not come from Paris. They were strengthened in their hostility by that half of humanity whose favor they chiefly sought, and who, as they had never experienced the miseries of the old attire, could never appreciate the comforts of the new. Men sneered at the costume without mercy, and branded it as hideous. As made and worn by many of its followers, it was certainly not beautiful: but had it been perfection itself, it would have utterly perished; for arrayed against it were the force of ignorance and of habit, and the persistent prejudices to which they give rise. Those who devised it had taken no pains to humor long-established tastes, or to induce a candid consideration of the advantages it would confer. While overrating the intelligence and courage of their followers, they had underrated the strength of their opponents. Before the ridicule that assailed it, its converts soon disappeared. A few clung to it resolutely: but they learned at last that the mental discomfort it brought to its singular adherents outweighed the physical comfort it gave; and they, too, went back, with a protest, to the old, detested garb. Thus the Bloomer costume has perished, and is remembered only as a tradition. Certain benefits it brought; but these are not what it sought to confer. A permanent reform of the dress of American women it has not effected; and it has, unquestionably, delayed its advent. So signal a failure has tended to discourage all subsequent efforts in the same direction, and has confirmed the thoughtless in their servile copying of foreign models.

But, had the costume succeeded in establishing itself as our permanent and recognized dress, it would not have rendered further reform unnecessary. The improvements it made, though conspicuous and important, were superficial. It simplified the clothing, lessened its weight, and gave freedom to the limbs; but certain pernicious features were retained. So long as the trunk of the body is girded in the middle by bands, with too little clothing above and an excess of it below, so long will the greatest evil of our present dress remain untouched.

Notwithstanding the lessons of the past, many still fancy that the object desired can be reached by a short and easy path. When dress-reformers seek for some wise and sure method of advancing their work, they meet advisers who say: "Fashion is the one powerful ally whom you should strive to gain: concentrate your efforts upon her; hunt her to her mysterious lair, — to that secret haunt beyond the seas, where, in busy silence, this frivolous Hecate brews the deadly potions she forces to our lips. There, convert her to your views, and the cause is won. Since we must all obey her behests, it behooves us to see that they are the behests of knowledge and of common sense."

To which we reply, Fashion is too fickle to be a valuable coadjutor in any work. Continual change is necessary to her very existence; and the costumes she imposes, however acceptable and good, can be but the whims and vagaries of an hour. To intrust vital principles to her is to write them upon the sand. Neither is she as despotic as she may seem. Her mandates reflect the wishes of her subjects; and, when we rail against her, we rail against a secondary cause. If she deserves opprobrium from us, it is because we force her to accede to our demands. She stoops to conquer the American market. At home, in Paris or Berlin, she amuses herself with the invention of ever-fresh absurdities of style; but they are for duchesses and queens, whose daily lives are of little value to the world or to themselves, and who can afford to give their time to the display of costly follies. We are a nation of earnest workers and of plain republicans; yet no absurdities that she conceives for others are absurd enough for us. We bid her send to our shores only her last and wildest conceits, and to add to them an extra touch. If she has delicate fabrics, we wish to wear them in our changeable climate; we require her to lengthen our trains, that we may drag them, on hurried errands, through unswept streets; to load our skirts with ornament, that we may bind them about our feeble frames; and to pinch and plait the slender bodices in which we do housework, tend shop, and lift unruly children. Fashion exclaims, "*Mon Dieu!* what glorious creatures these Americans are! They abound in money, and they adore my caprices. I must give them their hearts' desire!"

It is not against her power that we should strive, for she is more catholic in taste than her devotees, and more concessive to the requirements of reason. She now offers us good styles as well as bad; and that we adopt the bad rather than the good is not because of any inexorable necessity against which we hopelessly contend, but because, of our own free will, we prefer the worst that she can devise.

Moreover, she controls but a small portion of the domain of dress. The worst evils we experience are beyond her power to affect. It is for her to modify the outer costume, and to vary its countless details; but with the abiding and essential structure of the whole attire she has nothing to do. And what are a few ruffles more or less, a fitful change in the trifles of finish and trimming, to the inequalities of temperature, the burdens and the compressions, which our dress in every one of its many forms must inflict? They are but mint, anise, and cummin, compared with the weightier matters of physical laws perpetually broken by an established and unvarying style of senseless underwear, which has been handed down from generation to generation, and which we have all accepted from our mothers and grandmothers as the legacy of Fate, asking no questions as to its utility, and dreaming of nothing else as possible.

What is needed, then, is not to assail Fashion, but to teach Hygiene, — to awaken women to a consciousness of the injuries that follow the wearing of their present garments, and to demonstrate that it is in their power so to modify this tight, heavy, and complicated style of apparel as to increase the strength, ability, and happiness of themselves and of their children. Only through a general indifference to Nature's laws has a steady adherence to suicidal fashions been possible in the past. To remove such indifference should be the primal endeavor of any reformers who desire to lay the foundations for a broad and beneficent work.

In accordance with these views, the Association, of which mention has been made, took measures, early in the present year, for the public delivery of a series of free lectures to women, concerning the structure of their dress, and the important natural laws with which it conflicts. From a belief that no views would be so intelligent, and no words so effective, as those of experienced female physicians, a number of regularly educated and able members of the medical profession were selected, and urged to speak upon this theme. Most of them were personally unknown to the members of the Association; and all were chosen solely on account of their manifest fitness for the task. One has been for thirty years a well-known and successful practitioner, and during that period has had a wide acquaintance with the physical sufferings of her sex. Another is President of the Ladies' Physiological Institute, — a large and honorable society, —

and for a long time has taken charge of an important dispensary at the North End. Two are regular professors, and one a lecturer, in the Medical Department of the new Boston University; and all are practising physicians of good repute. The invitation extended to them they accepted without hope of recompense, and simply from a benevolent desire to stay the tide of misery and weakness which they are daily called upon to observe.

The lectures were not intended to be a connected course, but a series, where all should be kindred in scope, and each one complete in itself. There was, therefore, no assignment of any special topic to any special lecturer; nor did the lecturers hold any consultation beforehand, either together or with the Association, as to what should be said. The general theme assigned was "Dress, as it affects the Health of Women;" and the physicians were left to advance whatever assertions and opinions might seem to them good. Those for whom they spoke had no hobbies to present, no theories to uphold: their purpose was simply to obtain such a public presentation of facts concerning the dress of women as should command attention and induce reform. Thus the papers, when read, were as fresh to them as to any of the audience.

The entire freedom of expression which this plan secured might have been supposed to result in a wide dissimilarity of views. But, as if with intentional concurrence, these several physicians, of different experience, education, and schools, agreed, not only in general statements, but in the specification of the minutest details; and these statements were also in perfect unison with the conclusions to which the Association had previously been led.

The plan upon which the series had been given, and the uniformity of belief which it developed, implied, of course, some repetitions; but these were to be welcomed as evidences of the truth of what was said. It had not been the aim of the speakers to propound startling facts or singular opinions, but, without technical terms or learned speculation, to bear such plain, direct testimony to a few vital truths as should carry conviction to the minds of their hearers. Judging by the crowded and eager audiences that assembled to hear them, and the inquiries and endeavors subsequently put forth in the cause of reform, these efforts to benefit others met with a cordial and earnest response.

The claims of the physiologist were of such surpassing importance, that only one lecture in the series was devoted to the need of reform from an æsthetic point of view. In the closing paper, considerations of beauty, economy, and fitness received some recognition.

For women who are already convinced of the evils of their present dress, and who desire to provide for themselves a better, an Appendix has been prepared, in which will be found some explicit and practical suggestions in regard to the radical improvements that are capable of ready adoption to-day. It offers no regulation-suit for all to accept, irrespective of peculiar needs and preferences ; but, by defining clearly the principles upon which a proper dress should be constructed, and by presenting a variety of forms in which such principles may be embodied, it seeks to avoid those unnecessary limitations upon individual freedom which would be unwise if they were not futile.

TABLE OF CONTENTS.

Lecture	Page
I. By Mary J. Safford-Blake, M.D.	1
II. By Caroline E. Hastings, M.D.	42
III. By Mercy B. Jackson, M.D.	68
IV. By Arvilla B. Haynes, M.D.	98
V. By Abba Goold Woolson	124
Appendix	183
Index of Topics	255

DRESS-REFORM.

LECTURE I.

BY MARY J. SAFFORD-BLAKE, M.D.

THAT there is a growing discontent among women in regard to the clothes they wear, none can dispute, save those who having ears hear not. Whence arises this unrest, that, like a great billow, has broken over the land? Its origin can be distinctly traced to our growth: we have become women, and we desire to put away childish things.

When laws made by our forefathers are outgrown, when they are found to clog the wheels of progress, they are modified or rescinded, or they stand as dead letters upon the statutes. If, with enlarged spheres of action, the styles of dress imposed upon us by the *demi-monde* fashion-mongers of Paris, prove wholly insubservient to our needs, why accept them? Old-time superstitions are crumbling from under us in all directions. We begin to rejoice in the privilege, slowly accorded us, of thinking for ourselves, and of living true to our highest ideal of right. Possessed of ripened judgments and of justly matured opinions, we shall never be content so long as we are ruled in any direction by a merciless dictator. We have long since ceased to pay willing homage to this foreign despot, Fashion; and now, strengthened by the will and voice of many, the protest against her decrees has become so potent that we begin to rejoice in the hope of soon being able to consult our own individual tastes, needs, and conveniences in dress, as in other matters that pertain to our every-day life, without being a target for ridicule or for scorn.

Wherever the Gospel of Dress-Reform has been preached it has found waiting disciples. Encouraged to believe that the time had come for union of effort in this direction, an association of ladies was formed in Boston and in New

York a year since, which has been doing a good work in ferreting out the Protean forms of evil connected with dress, and in suggesting remedies for the same.

The association has not aimed at any radical changes in the externals of dress, save such as pertain to greater simplicity, to a convenient length of skirts, to less trimming, and hence to less weight. Much has been done to call attention to the modelling of undergarments, as well as to the material of which they are made. Several practical inventions for the suspension of clothing from the shoulders, for the lessening of the number of garments worn, and at the same time for the insuring of greater warmth, are the outgrowth of recent investigations. In order to have positive hygienic evidence brought to bear upon the ills entailed by improper dress, the association has arranged to have a series of lectures delivered in our city by women physicians, and it is the first of these which I have the honor of delivering to you this afternoon.

The subject has been canvassed from so many

points of view, that it would seem a hopeless task to add to it one thought more of interest, did we not realize that in this busy work-day world of ours, where each is hurried by the duties assigned him, it often occurs that the vital interests pertaining to self are overlooked. The man who lives within easy access of Niagara may never visit that phenomenon of nature; the grandest works of art are often little known by those born and bred near them, and so it may be in our familiar relation with self. We are prone to await a convenient season in which to acquaint ourselves with the laws of our being; and it not unfrequently happens that the fleshy tabernacle crumbles, totters, and falls before the mind has fully recognized the necessity of a harmonious relationship between soul and body.

One of the great blessings that the nineteenth century confers is that of associated effort. In the solving of social and scientific problems, we move in battalions; and when a victory is won, be it in Sitka or in Africa, the electric wire flashes an instantaneous announcement of it to the whole world. The boiling of Mother Watt's tea-pot, and the observation of it by her son James, enable us to-day to ride upon old ocean with the speed we do, and to bring within comfortable access our most distant shores. However insignificant the beginnings of effort seem, our vision is too limited to see in the dim vista of the future the final results.

In presenting to you some thoughts upon the subject of dress, than which I trust to convince you few are more vital, I do not desire you to accept my *ipse dixit* of right or of wrong; but I hope you will probe the facts presented, and, if they appeal to your common-sense and reason as truths, that you will heed them, not alone for your own good, but that your influence may go forth as a help and guide to others.

Converts to truth are variously affected: the scales fall from the eyes of one, and he says in his heart that which he sees is true; but he lisps his convictions to no one. Another preaches the glad tidings that, whereas he was blind, now he sees; but he acts as before. A third stands out like a bas-relief upon the flat surface of society, and lives the truth his soul has received. How stagnant would have become the streams of progress, if each believer had consulted his own individual comfort and ease! Boston might rock her cradle of Liberty to-day, and sing lullabies to her progeny of Freedom, with millions of fettered slaves in the land; but the conviction of wrong stamped itself upon the soul of a few, and they proclaimed it without thought of self-interest or of hindrance. There was principle to be maintained, and they moved on beneath its guidance till the bondmen were free.

Can my lady of leisure, who sits in her boudoir to-day with no imperative call to face the blinding snow or pelting rain, who can spend her mornings in dishabille, who can command carriage and horses to carry her dress-appendages,— can she look out from her damask-hung windows upon the hurried throng of business women, going early to the duties of the day, and returning late to their homes, and say there is no need of dress-reform?

If two women were to ascend Mount Washington, the one in a *porte-à-chaise* carried by four men, and the other on foot, would the former be justified in condemning the latter because she complained of the weariness and hindrance that the false burdens of fashion entail upon her?

In America there seems to be a general rage for a showy exterior, regardless of fitness of time, place, or circumstance. There are few lines of dress demarcation here to distinguish mistress from maid; and while the one enjoys a large share of favor, based, it may be, wholly upon externals, is it any wonder that the other apes her, even though it prove a hard-earned folly?

When I recently asked a young woman, who earns eight dollars per week, and pays seven dollars for her board and washing, what she thought would be the most effective way to help working girls into more practical, healthful, and economical modes of dress, her reply was, "Induce women of wealth and of position to adopt in their changes of style only those things that are comfortable and sensible, and we shall follow as they lead." It may be said that this is as absurd as if we should declare that because the poor cannot dwell in fine houses the rich shall not have them. I do not consider the two cases parallel. No doubt much of the extravagant luxury of modern palaces might well be dispensed with : but in matters of dress it is health and morals that we wish to elevate ; and no one has a right, measured by the highest law, to lead others astray, even by example. Offences must needs come, but woe unto him through whom they come! None can deny the moral side of this momentous question. If health and help ever reach us, it must come from above downwards. Women in high places, those upon whom are laid the weighty responsibilities of position, of wealth, and of influence, need but the strength of resolve and the force of action to stay this tide of extravagance and this perilously increasing physical degeneracy that over-dress is largely responsible for.

We scarcely fail in our daily peregrinations to

note the deference paid to fine clothes. The plainly dressed, hard-working woman enters a horse-car, laden perhaps with bundles, and she is left to stand; while the woman whose garments are modelled after the latest fashion-plate, whose jewels are adjusted to show themselves off to the most glaring advantage, is very sure to arouse the latent gallantry in some male heart, and this secures her a ready seat. He may find that good clothes and good breeding are not counterparts, for his courtesy may not receive the simple acknowledgment of "Thank you, sir."

Men are excellent theorizers upon the absurdities of dress; but when a practical application of their theories is made by their wives, daughters, or sisters, few are found brave enough to stand by and encourage these ladies to wear only such garments as are conducive to health and comfort.

Who that listened last winter to the painful cough of a celebrated prima donna upon the operatic stage could have failed to condemn the unjust demands of custom, which compelled that artist to trail behind her, as a graceful appendage, yards of soiled satin, thus rendering every movement that should have been one of freedom and of grace most painfully labored and affected? While her uncovered body was exposed to the prurient eyes of the world, at the risk of health and life, her stalwart male supporter, whose arm would have given a greater girth than her pinched waist, was dressed in thick velvet garments, and over these was thrown a loose, warm cloak. The next day the papers announced that the prima donna would be unable to appear owing to illness. Had she died, what pathetic sentiments would have been penned upon the physical frailty of woman!

That uniformity of temperature is desirable, is readily apparent from the fact that when any portion of the body becomes unduly heated for a prolonged period of time, congestion of the part is liable to follow; and when, on the other hand, a part is exposed to cold, the capillaries become contracted, the blood is thrown within, and any organ is liable to become engorged. The one which is weakened for any cause suffers most quickly and severely; and, unless an equilibrium of circulation is soon restored, inflammation follows. The myriad-mouthed pores of the skin, two thousand of which are found to occupy a square inch of surface, become closed, the tubuli leading from them become clogged, the carbonic acid the pores exhaled is retained, the oxygen they drank up is withheld, and the aeration of the blood then becomes wholly the work of the lungs. The frequently congested state of these organs during a cold is the result.

In woman's dress, from six to ten thicknesses are found, as a rule and not as an exception, to encase the thoracic region, while the lower extremities are covered, more frequently than otherwise, with but one thickness, and that of cotton. Under such circumstances, an effort to obtain proper warmth is usually made by adding an extra supply of skirts, although these garments contribute much more to pressure about the waist, weight upon the hips, and undue heat in the kidneys and abdominal organs, than to warmth in the lower extremities. But it is in these lower parts of the body that heat is most needed, because there the circulation of the blood is less active, and an under-current of air around them is apt to produce chills.

Let a woman step from a temperature of, perhaps, seventy degrees within doors, to zero without, and stand on the street corner five minutes for a car, while the breeze inflates her flowing skirts till they become converted into a balloon: the air whizzes through them and beneath them, and a wave of cold envelops the entire lower portion of the body. Then let her ride for an hour in a horse-car, with ankles wet from drabbled skirts, and exposed to a continual draft of air: of course her whole system is chilled through; and it cannot be otherwise than that a severe cold will follow as the penalty for such exposure.

A woman accompanied by her husband came to consult me on one of the dreariest days of last winter. Her teeth chattered with the cold; and you will not wonder at it, any more than I did, when I tell you that she had on cloth gaiter-boots, thin stockings, loose, light cotton drawers, two short skirts of flannel, a long one of water-proof, another of white cotton, an alpaca dress-skirt and an over-skirt. This made seven thicknesses, multiplied by plaits and folds, about the abdomen. Each of these skirts was attached to a double band; and thus the torrid zone of the waist was encircled by fourteen layers. All this weight and pressure rested upon the hips and abdomen; and the results were — what they must be, if this pressure has been long continued — a displacement of all the internal organs; for you cannot displace one, without in some way interfering with another. Here was this woman, with nerves as sensitive as an aspen-leaf to external influences, clad so that every breath of cold chilled her to the marrow, the neck and shoulders protected by furs, the hands and arms pinioned in a muff, the head weighted down by layers of false hair, and the legs almost bare; while her husband, the personification of all that was vigorous in health, was enveloped, as he told me, from head to foot in flannel. His every garment was so adjusted that it not only added to the heat generated by the body, but helped to retain it. I question whether that hale, hearty man would not have suffered twinges of neuralgia or of rheumatism, had he been exposed, as his wife was, to the severity of our atmospheric changes. Even in summer these changes are sudden and severe; and then men are usually clothed in woollen garments, only a trifle thinner and lighter than those worn in winter; while women are often decked in nothing but muslin, and are chilled by every sudden nor'-easter.

The soldiers of Austria were accustomed to retain their pantaloons about the hips by means of a leathern strap. Disease of the kidneys increased so alarmingly among them that especial attention was drawn to the subject; and it was decided that the closely buckled band about the loins was the cause of the evil. A decree then went forth making the adoption of suspenders imperative. It would have been wise if that imperial investigation had extended to the garments worn by women, and had led to a prohibition of the many bands and heavy weights that encircle and drag them down. The physical degeneracy of the mothers will leave its impress upon sons, as well as upon daughters; and in the end the national strength languishes under the weaknesses of inheritance.

The vigor of manhood in Austria is squandered in military service, and this throws much manual labor upon women. In Vienna, you will see in the early morning a rank and file of two hundred men and women awaiting the roll-call that shall apportion to each his or her labor for the day. Side by side with the men, women lay railroad iron, dig sewers, and carry up over steep ladders, on their heads or shoulders, brick and mortar for the laying of walls. Their dress, in length at least, is well adapted to the work assigned them: it reaches but little below the knee, and is there usually met by long boots. You see at a glance that the broad peasant waist has never been crowded into corsets, and you rejoice in the belief that it is free from the inward distortions that bone and steel are known to produce. But a fearful accident occurred in Vienna, while I was in the hospitals: a brick block of houses fell, killing and mangling several women who were employed in building them. "Now," I thought, as I entered the pathological room where a *post-mortem* examination was to be held upon them, "I shall once, at least, have an opportunity of seeing the internal organs of women normally adjusted." To my utter astonishment, it was quite the reverse. In one case, the liver had been completely cut in two, and was only held together by a calloused bit of tissue. Some ribs overlapped each other; one had been found to pierce the liver, and almost without exception that organ was displaced below the ribs, instead of being on a line with them. The spleen, in some cases, was much enlarged; in others, it was atrophied, and adherent to the peritoneal covering. The womb, of all internal organs the most easily displaced, owing to its floating position in the pelvis, and to the fact that it lies at the base, and is pressed upon by all above it, was in every instance more or less removed from a normal position.

I acknowledge that these peasant women were overburdened by hard labor; but many of the abnormal conditions I saw were dependent simply upon this fact, — that heavily quilted or home-spun skirts had been worn from childhood; and that these had always rested upon the hips, with each band snugly drawn about the waist and tied by strings.

It has been said that the injury caused by bands about the waist is obviated by wearing corsets beneath them. You need but a moment's reflection to see that this cannot be so. The pressure of the bands helps to adjust the steels and bones more closely to the yielding portions of the body. As no support is given to the corsets at the shoulders, and the skirts are not attached to them, they can furnish no relief whatever to the weight of garments resting upon the hips, and they add greatly to the unremitting downward pressure upon the abdominal organs.

Although these women did much hard work with nature so violated, still it stands to reason that they could not have had the same amount of strength and endurance that a normally organized body would have given them. It is always observed how much earlier they grow old than the men of their own rank; and this waste of force, this friction upon self, with the various added burdens they bear, is no doubt the cause.

Again, a terrible epidemic raged in the lying-in wards of Vienna, while I resided in the hospital of that city. In one week thirty women were consigned to their last resting-place. Here, also, I sought to make earnest research into the true relation to each other of the internal organs; and when I saw the condition of the majority of these poor women after death, I realized, as I could never have done without such opportunities, how danger and suffering increase, both for mother and child, in proportion as the former compresses and depresses her own body, and the embryo life it shields.

In my own country, the cases I have examined

after death have been limited in number, but nearly every one seen has revealed the same sad history. Chiefly through the courtesy of other physicians, I have had the opportunity to be present at the autopsy of several unmarried women. They were of the class not compelled to labor unduly, so that most of the abnormal conditions of the generative organs could be rationally accounted for only by improper dress. Whenever it was possible, I inquired into the habits of life and the modes of dress of the subject. In one girl, aged twenty-two, whose waist after death was so slender that you might almost have spanned it with united fingers, there was an atrophied state of all the glandular organs. It seemed to me possible, and even probable, that this condition had its origin largely in a continuous pressure upon that life-endowing nervous centre, the *solar plexus*, and upon the central glandular organs.

Recent experiments by a well-known physician of New York show conclusively that continual pressure brought to bear upon the stomach of animals causes their death more quickly than when applied to any other organ. The death of women occurring under the influence of anæsthetics has in many instances been traced to impeded circulation resulting from tight clothes.

However loosely corsets are worn, the steels and bones in them must adjust themselves to the various curves and depressions of the body, and must be felt, else the sure death that women so often declare would follow their abandonment would not be anticipated. As soon as the muscles give warning, by their weakness, that they are no longer adequate to the support of the body, it is high time they were given every chance to recuperate. Instead of this, we continue to hold them in immovable bondage. If the walls of a building were weak, we should expect only temporary aid from props ; but we should seek diligently for the cause of the weakness, and then turn all our efforts to remedy it. So it should be with our own muscular walls.

It does not require the foresight of a seer to diagnose a chronic case of tight lacing and of heavy skirts. You know in the main what the results must be: you know that when the abdominal muscular walls become inert, almost wasted, one of the important daily functions of the body is rarely, if ever, normally carried on. We might enumerate the ill results that follow; but these are only links in the long chain of disorders that have won the disgraceful appellation of women's diseases, when they should be termed women's follies. There has been no blunder in the formation of women: there would be harmony of action in each organ, and in the function assigned it, if Nature were not defrauded of her rights from the cradle to the grave.

The authorities whose opinions we most respect, because they are founded upon observation and research, and not upon blind prejudice, assure us that girls come out from the trying ordeal of coeducation unscathed. In mental calibre they are universally recognized as the peers of boys, now that they are beginning to have equal advantages with them for mental culture. Is it not, then, high time for the dawn of their physical development? But the only pleasurable and invigorating out-of-door exercise that girls have ever had has fallen into disfavor, because their dress was improper, and colds were contracted. Skating for girls seems doomed to be classed among the lost arts. I do not think that this one healthful exercise should be denied them, until it is tried under proper conditions.

A startling fact nearly precludes all gymnastic exercises in our schools : it is, that girls in their ordinary attire are so hampered in every ligament, joint, and muscle, that, in order to have perfect use and command of themselves for the brief space of an hour, this straight jacket, their clothes, in which they are encased sixteen hours of the day, must be wholly laid aside for looser and lighter raiment. If young ladies ride on horseback for exercise, as is done in some of our female colleges, what does it avail them, pinched and burdened as they are by their dress? If they row, it is under like conditions ; and the results are the same. What if our young men found it necessary to make an entire change in their apparel before they could drill, play base-ball, coast, or row? They would soon find it exceedingly irksome, and would seek, as girls have, their level of muscular inactivity.

With the cessation of school-life ends, for young women, the one hour per day of the chest-inflating, arm-extending, back-bending exercise that has been occasionally allowed them. If the dear graduate is so circumstanced that she must fall a victim to the epidemic rage of fashion, she will soon be called upon to struggle for days and weeks to keep her head above the Elizabethan ruff that threatens to swallow her up. But worse tortures than this await her. The thumb-screws of the inquisition might have been more painful to bear, but they certainly produced less harm than do the unyielding steels of her corsets, and the firm plates of metal attached as clasps to her belt, between which she is now cruelly pressed, and often so snugly that an impression of her fetters is indented into the flesh.

And what of her hair? Why, the poor girl has but just begun to recognize her own shadow on the side-walk, since the last sudden decree of fashion, when Simon says, "Thumbs up," and forthwith the rats, the mice, the luxuriant braids of hair and of jute rush to the top of her head, as if a pocket battery had been trifling with each. This new arrangement causes no little suffering. There is a great deal of pressure and heat on the top of the brain, and a physician is consulted. Mamma tells Æsculapius that once when her child was very young she played out in the sun, without her hat; that a sunstroke, or something like it, occurred; and that this affection is, very probably, the result of that exposure. "Most likely," responds Æsculapius; and he gives quieting powders. The scalp adapts itself, like all else in nature, to circumstances; but then a new fashion-plate arrives, and as with one fell swoop, at the command of "Thumbs down," the whole accumulation of braids, puffs, and curls drops from its lofty heights, and hangs suspended at the base of the brain.

Now the distress of the darling daughter has changed base: spinal meningitis is feared, and medical aid is speedily secured. Mamma can assign no cause for this new phase of suffering, unless it be that, some years before, her daughter fell on the ice. This time the pain proves so stubborn and severe that the Doctor is forced to suggest that the poor sufferer lay aside some of the superfluous weight of hair that has evidently caused more than a mere surface irritation. Vesicants would have been trifling to endure, compared with the mortification of being shorn, for the brief space of a few days, of those uncleanly false braids.

The causes of all our physical weakness are more assiduously sought for through a generation of grandfathers, than in false hair, kilt plaits, flounces, bustles, and corsets. But this pressure and weight of the daily dress would account for much of the physical prostration and enfeeblement of the women of our time. Many invalids, who are unable to lift a broom, habitually carry weights upon their heads and backs that the Humane Society would think cruel, if laid upon animals.

It is one of the sad reflections in connection with the absurdities and injuries of dress, that children are so early made to suffer by them. The weight and pressure of wide sashes, long, full bows, and over-skirts, are as heating and wearying, laid upon little backs, as are the various excrescences with which adult spines are freighted. The old saw, that "beauty unadorned is adorned the most," is never more aptly applied than to childhood. All that tends to rob this early age of its naturalness and simplicity deprives it of its greatest charm. It may be an old-fashioned whim, but it seems to me that the unsullied, unrumpled, high-necked apron, and the plain ungarnished calico of former days, made children more attractive than they can ever be when transformed, as they now are, by dictates of the latest fashion-plate, into miniature men and women.

And when the world is so full of good things to be done, which find no one to do them, may we not help to open the way by which the hewers of wood and drawers of water can aspire to higher conditions of labor? We say that our sewing keeps poor women employed; but is there no better way in which to exercise philanthropy than by dwarfing our souls and weakening our bodies that we may keep sempstresses at work? Very likely they could earn a much more healthful and quite as remunerative a livelihood by tilling the soil, or by entering into trades and professions. Is the American millionnaire, or the European princess, a model of Christian benevolence, when by her extravagant purchases she helps to keep thousands of pallid, half-starved girls bent over their lace-frames in the damp cellars of Belgium? Would it not be better to strive to render those women less miserable and dependent, by opening up to them more varied and healthful avenues of employment?

Time and money considered, nothing is more important in dress than the material of which it is made. A substantial, plain, elegant fabric carries on the face of it its own recommendation. Like a well-bred person, it is always presentable in any place and upon any occasion; while the flimsy stuff, however much ornamented, like a merely superficial character, shows its worthless origin; and the more you attempt to cover over its defects by gaudy externals, the more apparent they become.

And how much more economical and sensible is it to have one comfortable suit of clothes, adapted, in color, cut, and warmth, to our needs, than to possess a variety of garments, none worn enough to justify us in abandoning them, but all left on our hands when the season ends! The remodelling of such attire, which thus becomes a part of the next year's labor, really consumes more time, and gives more annoyance, than the making of wholly new garments.

I retain as a delightful memory an evening spent at the house of a German Professor in Berlin. There were rare minds gathered together from many lands, men and women whom one had known and prized from afar. The charming manner in which the *Frau Professorin* welcomed her guests left nothing to be desired. I do not know that any other than my American eyes took note, even, of her dress; certainly no one seemed to scrutinize it. But she was arrayed in a pearl-colored silk, which, as I afterward learned, had been her wedding gown, made fourteen years before. It had a long bodice, with small plaits at the waist and broad ones upon the shoulders; an open front, with lace under-kerchief; mutton-leg sleeves, closed at the wrist, with a frill of lace about them; and the skirt was short and full, and gathered upon the waist. Her hair, all her own, was gathered into a meagre knot behind.

I could but make an estimate then of the probable time she had saved from those fourteen years by wearing her gown as it was first made. I felt sure, taking into consideration the matching of material, the selection of trimmings, the confabs with dressmakers, that would have been necessary to keep the dress modernized in accordance with the changing demands of the mode, that months of precious time had thus been spared to the wearer, and peace of mind beyond computation. Who could tell but that those days, weeks, and possibly months, were what gave her the time, in part, to learn to converse fluently with her guests, as she did, in as many different languages as they represented?

In our great republican hive, the working-women — by which term I mean every woman with a decided employment, be it mental or manual (and, as civilization advances, there will be few others) — must, sooner or later, have the same privileges as regards dress accorded to them in our social circles that are granted now to men. If a woman is closely occupied during the day, it may be quite impossible, or at least very inconvenient, for her to lay aside her usual garb for the adornments of the evening. Her companion in work gives hair and coat a brush, sees to it that his linen is immaculate, and takes no further thought for the occasion, to which he is also invited.

And, little by little, people begin to expect consistency and fitness in the dress of women occupied in earnest work. An invalid said to me not long since: "For years, upon my couch, I have traced the footsteps of those who have taken a front rank in the march for freedom and truth. This winter, for the first time, I was enabled to listen to the voices of those whose sayings had become household words to me; and imagine my surprise to see Mrs. Blank's grand features set in a high ruff, with ear-rings in her ears, false braids towering upon her head, and her dress sweeping the platform! Why, to have seen William Lloyd Garrison in a *Louis Quinze* powdered wig, knee-buckles, and embroidered coat-tails, would not have surprised me more." Lucretia Mott would cease to be the treasured picture we carry in memory, were she divested of her simple, unchanging Quaker garb. Florence Nightingale would become common clay, instead of the angel of the hospital, were she to be represented to us in the ridiculous disfigurements of pannier, chignon, and leathern girdle with its string of dangling trinkets.

Let a high and holy purpose take possession of the soul, and the body becomes its willing subordinate. The world, so often blinded to its best interests, at last learns to recognize the worth of the aim, the value of the mind. Externals in time are lost sight of; and the individual is sought after for what she is and does, and not for the value of her diamonds, the rarity of her lace, and the quality of her velvet.

When medals and titles had been conferred by the majority of European nations upon Professor Opholzer of Vienna, the Emperor, Francis Joseph, remembering that a prophet was not without honor save in his own country, informed the revered professor that a medal awaited his acceptance. A few days after, the old professor came to his clinic in the early morning as usual, followed by a swarm of disciples. When he had finished his wearisome hours of instruction at the bed-side of the sick, he drove to the Imperial Palace. Conceive of the horror of the finely dressed usher, when he beheld the professor come in his work-day suit to enter into the august presence of his sovereign. No, that could never be. A dress-suit, white neck-tie, and white gloves were indispensable to the receiving of a medal. The professor replied that the duties of his profession precluded such ceremony; that, if His Majesty desired it, he would send his good clothes to him, but that he had no time to wear them. He drove away, and never returned to receive the honor that his dress-suit might have won for him.

So long as women are subordinate to the clothes they wear, so long will social intercourse be the prattling, superficial thing it everywhere is, and so long will parties and receptions literally mean nothing but exhibitions of wearing apparel. Communion, Easter, and Baptismal costumes! Alas for the example of the meek and lowly Master!

We must have something of the stability in our styles of dress that characterize the clothes of men. It seems to me that fifteen minutes in the spring, and fifteen in the fall, must suffice for a man to provide himself with all the clothes he needs for comfort and for adornment. He is allowed to smile at the devices of his tailor, and to hold to old fashions till they are threadbare; but let a woman be five years behind the style, and where in society is there a niche for her to fill?

At every National, State, and County Exposition we ought to have a dress department, where the best materials will be shown, and where styles will be discussed from a hygienic, æsthetic, and economic point of view. Then we shall begin to have doctors of dress; and there will be specialists in the profession, those who will recommend to us colors and textures, those who will see to it that we are so well dressed that no one can tell what we wear, and so comfortably attired that self and clothes blend into an harmonious whole. Then there will be no meteoric flashes of style, only a slight modification in the cut and fit, when, in the course of human events, a change of garments becomes a necessity.

In that good time coming, the aurora of

which it is hoped is now seen above the horizon, nothing will astonish and grieve us more than to reflect upon the life and energy we here squandered in clinging to that worst form of barbarism in our dress, the trailing skirts. Shorn of them, we are told, we should be bereft of our grace, our loveliness, our womanliness. It would seem as if any one, however blinded by the customs of his time, might see the absurdity of a nation of intelligent women allowing themselves, under protest, to be converted into city, town, and country scavengers, without thanks or the recompense of admiration from those whose approval is most to be desired. For women who go thus hampered, there can never be one step free from filth and annoyance of some kind, unless the skirts are clutched and held up by main force. Even at summer resorts, by the sea-side and in mountain places, where people flee from all that is wearisome to the spirit and to the flesh, even here only an occasional woman is found brave enough to remove this objectionable feature of her dress, and to let the poor, overburdened body become really free. When she does follow the dictates of her own conscience, her friends often feel it incumbent upon them to reward her good sense by saying, "She always was peculiar." The young miss who may tower, perhaps, head and shoulders above her seniors, does not shock the hyper-sensitive world by the shortness of her gown, and the exposure of her feet and ankles. But let her grow in years, though not in stature, and she becomes a monster in the eyes of the public, if she insists upon retaining the freedom of movement that her short dress formerly insured.

There really seems no prescribed limit to the height to which skirts may be lifted in walking, if only the wearer is hung round about with clogging folds from which she can never free her hands without paying the penalty of wet and mud-bedraggled hems. Holding on to her draperies as if for dear life, she may raise them to the knees, and her style of clothing is tolerated with complacency. But let it be known and seen that the dress is hung so as never to come below the tops of the boots, and that the limbs are properly and decently covered with leggins which fit closely, or with Turkish trousers fastening at the ankle, and what fears are harbored for the appearance and the morals of women! Instead of such attire being ugly, it can be made most tasteful and becoming. All travellers, I think, express only admiration for the short costumes universally worn by the peasantry of Europe. There, some individuality in taste is exercised, and the result is a pleasing picturesqueness in the dress of the people. With us, at present, the requirements of beauty are wholly disregarded by the adoption of styles unsuited in every way to their wearers.

There seems a dread suspicion in the minds of some that women have no other aim in their desire for dress-reform than that of adopting the hideous style of clothes worn by men. I see little besides the durability of the material and the lightness and warmth of their clothing which is worthy to be adopted by us.

I cannot believe that the earnest, thinking

women of America will ever cease to demand it as a right and a privilege to dress so that they can meet unfettered the duties that they assume or that are thrust upon them. Now, health, strength, and energy are exhausted in the friction that results from carrying superfluous burdens, — burdens which have been handed down to them from an age when women were passive instead of active members of society. The trailing and *décolleté* dress of the *salon* is historically one of the relics of the period of lust, when women were shut out of the kingdom of thought, and were linked with men only in bonds of sensuality. When men have higher estimates of women, and women more self-respect, their loveliness will not be determined by bare arms and shoulders, and by trailing silks, any more than the manliness of man is now by the broadcloth he displays.

Before closing, let us briefly recapitulate features that ought to be introduced into any rational dress-reform. The under-garments should suffice, in the quantity and quality of their material, to give suitable warmth to the entire body; and the distribution of this warmth should be as equable as possible. To facilitate speed in dressing, and to obviate the necessity for the many bands now worn about the waist, unite in one suit vest or waist and the lower garment. Let no weight whatever rest upon the hips; and if the shoulders rebel against their burdens, lighten the weights they bear. Let the stockings be suspended, by means of an elastic band depending from the vest or from the union garment, if you would find no marks of impeded circulation upon the limbs. Let the stockings in winter be woollen, if you find them comfortable; but if not, then let them be fleece-lined, — the heavier, the better. Leggins are never to be dispensed with in this climate during the winter season. Be sure to have the soles of your shoes broader than your feet, and the heels low and broad, if you would walk with ease, and avoid corns and bunions. To insure warm feet in winter, and not overheated ones in summer, wear heavy soles the year round. The higher the tops of the boots, the warmer the ankle, provided they are so loose that the circulation is free. If your work permits it, have the material of which your dress is made firm and enduring. If occupied in housework, washable material is desirable, not necessarily calico, so thin and cold for winter, but some serviceable woollen stuff. If a constant attendant upon the sick, there must be no rustle to your garments, and they must be frequently changed and washed. If you would not carry contagion from the sick room, do not wear false hair; for it may become impregnated with disease germs. If you would avoid many nervous affections, neuralgia, and sick headache, if you would keep the scalp clean and free from disease, then do away with that mass of dead material, false hair. It calls to itself floating impurities, and gives only heat, weight, and weariness to the head; while it destroys the beautiful outline of the head, and all symmetry of proportion between its size and that of the body. If you would retain a fair skin, and have the face free from pustules, let the blood flow unimpeded to every part. Keep the skin active by the use of pure water, and avoid the "Balm of a Thousand Flowers," and all cosmetics, under whatever alluring names presented. If you cover your face with veils, you may save your pallid complexion, but you will injure your sight. I have the best authority that the world has ever known for saying this. Dr. Von Grafe, the lamented oculist of Berlin, whose memory is revered in every land, told me he believed one of the prolific causes of amaurosis, — that disease in which specks float before the eyes, — among women, was the wearing of spotted lace veils; and of near-sightedness among children, the wearing of any veils. So, as you prize the precious gift of sight, avoid the things that may weaken it, or deprive you of it altogether.

Finally, if women would live true to the highest ideal for which they were created, and would measure their lives by noble deeds, let them make for the soul imperishable garments, and give only such thought to the clothing of the perishable body as will suffice to render it strong and efficient for carrying out the soul's behests.

LECTURE II.

BY CAROLINE E. HASTINGS, M.D.

LADIES, — I come before you this afternoon to speak upon the subject of dress-reform. It is a subject which is engaging the attention of many at the present time ; and its agitators, feeling encouraged with here and there a convert, have conceived the idea of presenting it before different audiences, hoping to rouse the common-sense of women to come to the rescue, and to aid them in overthrowing the tyranny of the despotic and ever-changing goddess, Fashion.

To me the service which this ruler demands of her subjects is simply appalling ; and nothing, I think, could make me more miserable, mentally or physically, than to be obliged to adopt the costume of a fashionably dressed woman. On the other hand, I suppose nothing would make one of Fashion's devotees more miserable mentally

— mind, I do not say physically, in this case — than to be obliged to dress as simply as do some of the dress-reformers.

I shall endeavor to demonstrate to the eye that the present style of woman's dress does interfere with her best health; and I hope the reasons for my statements will seem to you so conclusive that some, at least, may be won from the error of their ways. To this end, I ask your attention to certain facts concerning the construction of the human body. And, before going any farther, let me say that there are probably, in this audience, many who have attended excellent lectures upon that and kindred subjects, and who are therefore well acquainted with both anatomy and hygiene. To such, a great deal of what I shall say will be as familiar as household words. But is not this true of any reform? Who can reveal any thing new upon the subject of Temperance? And yet the discussion on that theme holds the attention of the public mind, however often it may be repeated. We have but one story to tell; and what we mean to do is to tell this story over and over, till women shall listen and heed the warning.

In a printed report of the lecture given last Wednesday, it was stated that "the treatment of the subject thus far had been more an elaboration of the injurious effects of the present styles of dress than of what dress-reform should be." I do not understand the object of these lectures to be to propose a certain style of attire to be adopted as a uniform; but rather to arouse the minds of women to the fact that the present styles of dress are injurious, and to tell them wherein and how these styles act injuriously, leaving each woman to adopt for herself any external costume or style that she may prefer.

We only insist that the attire shall be so constructed as to hang from the shoulders; that it shall be of sufficient waist-measure to allow a continual full expansion of the chest, and of a length that shall prevent the dress from doing the work of the scavenger. I say we aim first to convince women that there is need of a reform in dress; and we believe that, when they are once thoroughly convinced of this, they will bring about a style suited to the wants and the comfort of the body, — perhaps by carrying out an idea suggested in the first lecture of this course, viz., that "at every National, State, and County Exposition, we ought to have a dress department, where the best material may be shown, and where styles, from a hygienic, æsthetic, and economic point of view, may be discussed." The demand itself will furnish the means, and show us the way. Our duty is to create the demand.

First, then, we will consider the bony framework of the body; and I am fortunate in being able to show you a specimen this afternoon. Some of the bones enclose cavities, — as, for instance, the ribs, which enclose the thoracic cavity; and again the hip-bones, as they are familiarly called, which, with the lower part of the spine, form a cavity known as the pelvic cavity. Between these two cavities lies another, which has no bony walls, only walls of flesh.

The thoracic cavity, as I have said, is formed by the ribs, twenty-four in number, twelve on each side, with the breast-bone in front, and the spinal column behind. To the spine the ribs are joined by strong ligaments; but they are finished out and attached to the breast-bone by means of cartilage, with the exception of the two lower, which are attached only to the spine. As these are not attached to the breast-bone, they are called floating ribs. The cartilaginous attachments permit the cavity thus enclosed to be expanded to a great extent, provided their elasticity is not interfered with by some contrivance supposed to be an improvement upon the original plan. When these cartilages become ossified, as they sometimes do, from disease or old age, the ribs are fixed in position, and the chest can no longer dilate. This is not considered an advantage, but a misfortune. The same result, if it follows the wearing of a garment, occasions no concern; but I can see little difference between the two evils. I believe that any lady, young or old, must experience serious

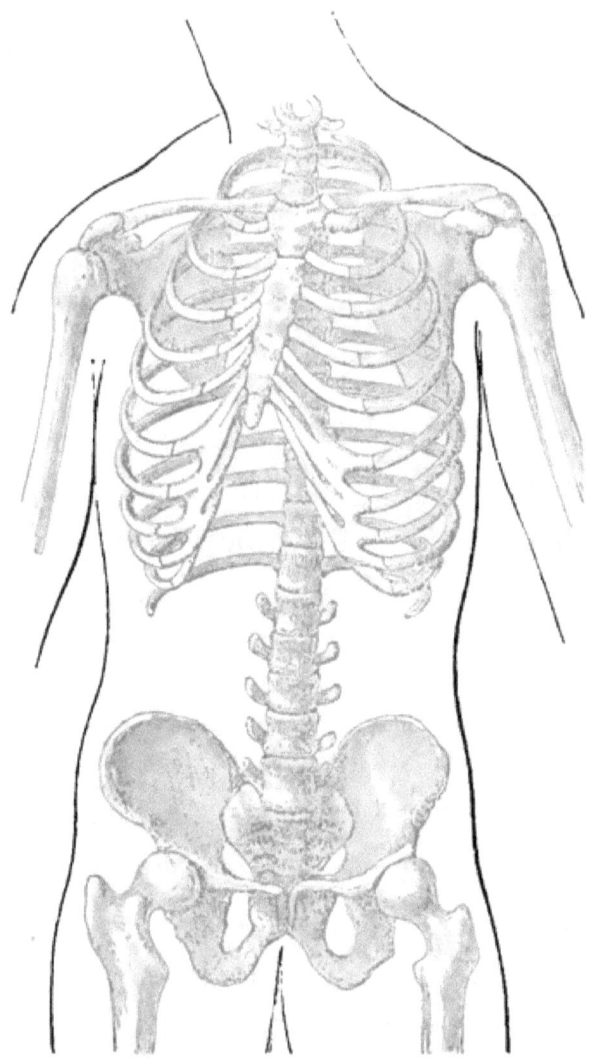

BONY FRAMEWORK OF THE BODY.

injury when she interferes with one of Nature's wise designs by compressing these twenty-four ribs to such an extent that the cartilages in which they terminate cannot act. What difference does it make whether these ribs expand or not, you may ask. The difference between ease and disease. The form of the ribs is more readily changed than that of any other bones of the body; for their situation is such that the constant pressure of the clothing above them day after day needs to be but slight to bend them downwards and inwards. Well, you say, what if they are bent downward and inward? what harm is done? It is an old saying that Nature abhors a vacuum. There is no unoccupied space in the body; and to render any part of it smaller than Nature designed is to cause the organs occupying that part to diminish in size, or to crowd together one upon another. In either case, Nature's processes are sadly interrupted. It does not require any great pressure to lessen the capacity of the thoracic cavity, provided the process be begun in early life.

Snugly fitting dresses worn from childhood till the age of eighteen or twenty will accomplish the result; but, as if to make assurance doubly sure, the mother buys a compress, which she clasps around the body of her little girl while yet the bones are in their most yielding state. And no wonder the girl of sixteen or eighteen thinks she cannot live without her corsets. The muscles, never having been allowed to do the work of supporting the spinal column and abdominal organs, refuse to come up to the full measure required of them at a moment's notice, and, as a natural consequence, the young lady feels all she expresses when she says, "It seems as though I should drop to pieces without my corsets."

Within this thoracic cavity of which I have been speaking are contained the vital organs,— viz., the lungs and heart,— called vital because an entire suspension of their functions for a few minutes will result in death.

The lungs, which are the essential organs of respiration, are composed of tubes, blood-vessels, and air-cells; and these are held together by a thin connective tissue. The tubes are branches of the trachea or wind-pipe. These branches divide again and again, as a tree divides into branches and twigs, till they become too minute to be seen with the naked eye. At the utmost extremity of each of these twigs may be seen little bladders or air-cells, which receive the air as it comes through the tubes. It is estimated that there are 600,000,000 of these air-cells in one pair of lungs. The blood-vessels coming from the heart divide and subdivide, and finally form a network around each one of the air-cells. All the blood in the body passes through the lungs once in five minutes, to be oxygenized. The oxygen is taken with every breath into these air-cells, and is given off to the blood through the membranes of the air-cells and the blood-vessels. The blood in turn gives up its carbon, and that which upon entering the lungs was a purplish hue becomes a bright cherry color. Thus vitalized, it is returned to the left side of the heart, to be sent out all over the body, carrying life and health to every part. Situated between the lungs is that hollow muscular organ, the heart; and below them is the liver, the greater part of which lies upon the right side, and extends downward, in its normal position, to about the lower border of the tenth rib. The diaphragm is the internal breathing muscle; and it acts a very important part in the process of respiration. It is attached in front to the lower portion of the breast-bone; on either side, to the inner surfaces of the cartilages and bony portions of six or seven lower ribs; and behind, to that part of the spinal column known as the lumbar region.

Now as to the action of the diaphragm. It modifies to a great extent the size of the chest above it, and the position of the thoracic and abdominal viscera below. During inspiration, the cavity of the chest enlarges in a vertical direction nearly two inches, and the greater part of this increase is due to the descent of the diaphragm. I have been thus minute in this description for a reason that will appear later.

Let us compress the chest by putting a bandage around the ribs: draw it tight, and what is the effect? You can hardly find breath to say, "Oh! I cannot breathe;" you grow red in the face; the head seems ready to burst. What is the trouble? Why, you have so compressed the lungs that the air cannot pass into the air-cells, and you are in a state of asphyxia, and this means a suspension of the respiratory process.

Let us look for a moment at the result of such a suspension when it becomes entire. You will remember about the network of blood-vessels surrounding the air-cells. A complete suspension of respiration causes a retardation or stoppage of the circulation through this network. Now the blood, arrested in the lungs, ceases to reach the heart in sufficient quantities to support the action of that organ, and the phenomena of life are suspended. In order that the blood may pass through the pulmonary veins into the left heart, it must be changed from venous to arterial blood; that is, the blood which is charged with carbonic acid upon arriving at the lungs must give off this poison, and at the same instant receive the oxygen, which has been brought into the air-cells in the air we have inhaled. But the pressure we have applied has prevented this change from venous to arterial blood, by cutting off the supply of oxygen ; the blood cannot return to the left side of the heart, and the lungs cannot receive any more from the right side of the heart ; neither can the right heart receive any further supply from the veins which usually empty their contents into it ; and consequently we have a state of congestion all over the system. If this pressure should be kept up from two to five minutes, death would be the result.

The chest of a pugilist was so much compressed by an attempt to take a plaster cast of his body in one piece that all action of the muscles of respiration was prevented. As he was unable to speak, the danger of death became imminent ; but his situation was discovered in time, and his life saved.

I have been describing the consequence of a complete suspension of respiration, which is death in from two to five minutes. Has it occurred to you that there is one article of woman's dress so constructed that, when clasped around the waist, it applies this pressure, — not to the extent of instant death indeed, but yet to such an extent that those who wear it live at

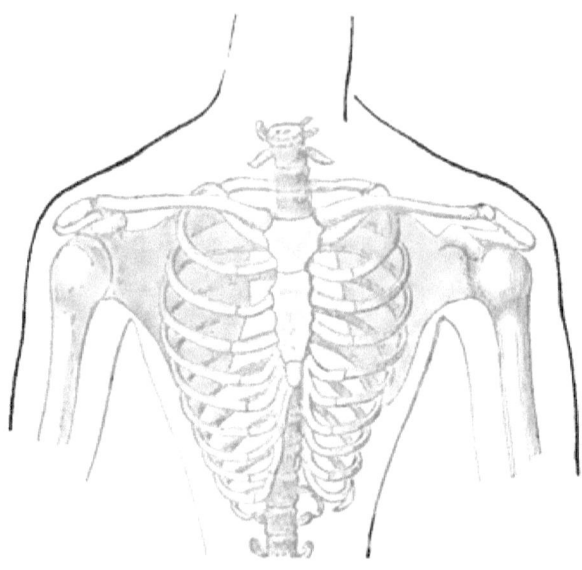

a dying rate? The corset is the name of this instrument of human torture. So far as I am able to learn, no one takes to corsets naturally, and it is only after hours of suffering that one becomes able to endure them without pain, — I mean, of course, if by good fortune one has lived to the age of thirteen or fifteen without them. But now-a-days children's corsets are for sale, and almost as soon as the little girl is able to walk these are put upon her.* Too young to enter

* A few days ago, I stepped into a large corset manufactory that is carried on by a woman. I told her I was interested to know what women and children wear in this line, and asked to see her wares from the least unto the greatest. She began by showing me the tiniest article I ever saw in the shape of a corset, saying that was for babies. Then she brought forward another grade, and still another, and so on, till I think she must have shown me fifteen or twenty different-sized corset moulds, in which she runs the female forms that get into her hands. She informed me that all the genteel waists I should meet on the fashionable streets of the city she made; that the mothers brought their daughters in infancy to her, and that she passed them through the whole course of moulds till they were ready for the real French corset, when she considered them finished and perfect.

Yesterday I visited the first class in one of our city girls' grammar schools, consisting of forty-two pupils. I had five questions on a slip of paper, that I asked permission of the teacher to put to the girls : —

First. — "How many of you wear corsets?"

Answer. — "Twenty-one." I asked them to stretch their arms as high as they could over their heads. In every instance it was hard work, and in most cases impossible, to get them above a right angle at the shoulders.

Second question. — "How many of you wear your skirts resting entirely upon your hips, with no shoulder-straps or waists to support them?"

Answer. — "Thirty."

Third question. — "How many wear false hair?"

Answer. — "Four."

a protest, and too young to be heeded if she should, she grows up accustomed to the pressure, and scarcely realizes the change from children's to ladies' corsets.

Just here, perhaps, you are recalling the position of the lungs, and saying that corsets do not encroach upon the region occupied by those organs, and therefore cannot compress them, and that all my charges fall to the ground. Not so fast, my dear girl! Please to recall the diaphragm, and its attachments to the lower part of the breast-bone and to the inner surfaces of five or six lower ribs, and then tell me if the pressure applied by corsets does not fall directly over this region.

> Fourth question. — "How many wear tight boots?"
> Answer. — "None" (which I doubted).
> Fifth question. — "How many do not wear flannels?"
> Answer. — "Eighteen."

I went across the hall to a boys' class, corresponding in grade, consisting of forty-four pupils. I asked for the number of boys without flannels, and found only six.

Of course one hundred per cent were without corsets, or weight upon hips, or tight boots, or false hair. Every boy could raise his arms in a straight line with his body, as far as he could reach, with perfect ease. — From a published Paper entitled *Corsets* vs. *Brains*, by Louise S. Hotchkiss.

For a complete filling of the air-cells, the cavity of the chest must be enlarged, in order to accommodate an increased expansion of the lungs; and I have shown you that this increase in the size of the cavity is due, in a great measure, to the depression of the diaphragm. Now, if you have compressed the ribs and cartilages so much that they cannot act, the diaphragm remains nearly or quite motionless, the cavity is smaller than is requisite for a complete filling of all the air-cells. a part of the blood is not oxygenized, and the system suffers just in proportion to the amount of carbonic acid retained in the blood.

"But I do not wear my corsets too tight," every lady is ready to answer. I never yet have been able to find a woman who did, if we accept her own statement; and yet physicians are constantly called upon to treat diseases which are aggravated, if not caused, by wearing corsets. Nature is long suffering, and for a time yields her rights so quietly that we do not realize how we are imposing upon her. But a day of reckoning will surely come, perhaps too late. You do not wear your corsets too tight, you say. Tell me, then, why they unclasp with a snap, and why you involuntarily take a long, deep breath when you unclasp them.

If you will allow me, I will explain why you take that long, deep breath. All day the blood has been seeking to enter the blood-vessels of the lungs in a greater quantity than they were able to receive on account of the pressure upon them. Now the pressure is off; and the blood, no longer obstructed, rushes into the network of blood-vessels surrounding the air-cells, and instantly there is a call for oxygen to take the place of the carbonic acid contained in it. Involuntarily we answer this call with a deep breath, and a complete filling of the air-cells. In a moment equilibrium is restored; the blood flows into the lungs more steadily, and an easy respiration is then sufficient to supply the demand for oxygen.

But I have hinted at diseases produced and aggravated by this continued pressure. For instance, the obstruction of pulmonary circulation may and does cause enlargement of the left ventricle of the heart, as well as congestion of brain, liver, and kidneys.

Nearly a year ago a young lady complained to me that she was troubled with palpitation of the heart, at times quite seriously so. A glance was sufficient to show me that she wore corsets, and that they were drawn to the last fraction of an inch. I told her she was injuring herself; and, that I might prove it, induced her to let me measure the corsets as she was wearing them. I found they measured just twenty-two inches. I then put the tape-measure around her waist, and, holding it loosely between thumb and finger, asked her to fill her lungs. She did so, and the measure drew out to twenty-six inches. So you can readily see that she was sacrificing health to a fancied style of beauty. I am sorry to say that she would not change her habit, and I have since known this same young lady to get another to hook her corsets for her, because they were so small that she could not possibly bring them together.

I am very glad to be able to give you an instance which proves, on the other hand, that there is still some sense left among women. A young lady came to me quite out of health, and with symptoms of weakness of the lungs. Among other remedies I prescribed the leaving off of corsets, which advice she was willing to receive and adopt. She became very much better; and I believe a greater part of the improvement was due to the giving up of corsets, aided by a few weeks in the country, where the lungs were at liberty to take in God's sweet air without hindrance. About six months after, she wished to attend a wedding reception, and thought she would put on the corsets, just for the evening. To use her own words, she was in agony till she could get home and take them off, thus proving what I have before stated, that women do not take to corsets naturally.

I think I have given you good reasons why you should not wear corsets; and now let me suggest in their place a waist cut to fit the form, a basque waist, with a strong band stitched upon the skirt or lower part. Upon this band sew five or six buttons, and in the bands of all the skirts work button-holes to correspond. You will then have all your clothes suspended from the shoulders without straps or tapes, which I have always found inconvenient from the fact that they will slip off from the shoulders. Having thus suspended your skirts to a loose, well-fitted waist, you not only allow plenty of room for the expansion of lungs, but you avoid any stricture about that part of the body situated between the thoracic and pelvic cavities, and which has only muscular walls. The stricture caused by bands about the waist when they are worn without corsets has been an argument in favor of the latter article of dress ; but the style of waist proposed will remedy this evil, while it accommodates itself to the needs of chest and lungs.

But why, if we leave the lungs free to act well their part, need we remove the weight of clothing from the hips ? This brings us to consider the pelvic cavity and its contents. This cavity is formed by the union of the two bones called in familiar language hip-bones with each other in front, and with the lower part of the spinal column behind. In the lower part of this cavity are situated the bladder and the uterus or womb. Above these organs are twenty-five feet of intestines lying loosely in the abdominal cavity, with no great amount of support from above. These lower organs are joined together by the folding over and around of the membrane called peritoneum, so that whatever displaces one will affect the others to a certain extent. There are some ligaments which hold them in position, but they will yield if too great or too long-continued pressure be exerted from above downwards. In this way some of the diseases peculiar to woman are brought about.

When the weight of clothing is supported only by the hips, it has a tendency to press down the intestines, and their weight must then fall upon the organs below. These, in their turn, are forced to yield. One of the rules for treatment of diseases of this nature laid down in the books is, "Remove all weight from the hips."

Well, having fastened your skirts in this way, make them as light as possible for the sake of the shoulders, lest you may overburden them. To this end, make the skirts as free from heavy trimmings as possible, and cut off the extra length that requires a facing of wiggin or leather to keep it tolerably clean. Do this with your walking dresses, at least; and then, having a broad, low heel upon your boot, a half day's shopping, or even a whole day's, may be accomplished with ease and comfort.

If you have cut off the train, you will be able to dispense with that other superfluity, the pannier, — I believe that is the name of the excrescence, — and which when worn bears upon a region that ought not to be subjected to heat or pressure. In the region which this article of dress covers, the kidneys are situated; and just below them, upon either side, large bundles of nerves make their exit from the spinal cord, and pass downward to the lower extremities. Any continued pressure over this region will tend to cause either a dormant condition of these nerves, or perhaps an irritation which will result in pain and lameness. A young lady of my acquaintance — who, because it is the fashion, feels herself obliged to wear one of these deformities — always suffers a severe pain in the hip as a penalty, and yet she must wear it when she goes out, for "how she would look without it!"

Will the time ever come when women will assert their rights in the matter of dress, — when each shall be free to adopt a style which allows the full and free use of all the powers, both physical and mental, with which God has endowed her? It need not necessarily be one that shall be noticeable for its oddity; it need not be one so closely resembling that of the masculine sex as to subject us to the charge of wishing to be men. I believe that about all I envy in man's apparel is the opportunity for pockets which it affords. These I would like.

Then there is a moral side to this question of

dress, which I do not propose to discuss at any great length, but I will mention it, and leave honest, conscientious minds to ponder and decide its value. Is it right for us to pay so much worship to dress? is it right to make it the criterion of respect and favor in the horse-car, in the church, at the party? So long as richly dressed women take precedence everywhere because they are richly dressed, so long will the tempter find it easier to secure his victim. Human nature is the same in all. Love of attention is as strong and legitimate in the girl who is obliged to earn her daily bread as in the girl whose father pays her bills. We all know the low wages received by the girls who wait upon us at the many stores throughout the city. These wages scarcely suffice, in many cases, to pay for room rent and for food! What, then, of clothes to wear? Oh, shame! upon men in this city, who, when the innocent girl pleads that the low wages offered will scarcely pay for living expenses and she demands "wherewithal shall I be clothed?" shame — yes, and God's wrath

— upon those who answer, "You can find some friend who will give you these for your company." I am not imagining a case now, but telling you a fact. Then the struggle grows hard: the desire for dress for the sake of the attention, not to say the common civility, which is accorded to it, becomes stronger; and, too often the temptation is greater than she is able to bear.

Now who is to blame? The girl, certainly; but are not we, who allow so much to depend upon dress, somewhat — yes, greatly — responsible for the snare which has caught her young feet? Can we not help her by adopting a style of dress that shall not put such a difference between the appearance of the rich and the poor?

There is, in the future of us all, a day when all these outward adornings must be laid aside, and when we must give an account unto Him who has said, "Whoso causeth one of these little ones that believe in me to offend, it were better that a millstone were hanged about his neck, and he be cast into the sea;" and again, "Inasmuch as ye did it unto one of the least of these, ye did it unto me."

Ladies, — I thank you for your presence here, and for your attention during the hour. I trust that the seed I have attempted to sow has fallen upon honest minds, and that some of it may spring up and bear fruit a hundred-fold.

LECTURE III.

BY MERCY B. JACKSON, M.D.

LADIES, — We propose to speak to you this evening upon dress in its relations to health, its uses and abuses.

Having observed the great evils that result from the present modes of dress, and perceiving that a fundamental change is needed in this respect, if woman's vigor and usefulness are not to become seriously impaired, we have been induced to speak to you, well knowing our inability to treat the subject in a manner worthy of its importance. Relying upon your indulgence, we would ask attention to the few thoughts which we have thrown together during the brief intervals of a busy professional life, hoping they may not prove wholly uninteresting and useless.

We are living in an age of progress, when ideas are asserting their right to rule, and are taking the sceptre from brute force, which has so long held sway. Consequently, women are awaking to a consciousness of powers unused, and of fetters on mind and limb which have hitherto prevented them from doing their share of the world's work. They see that these obstructions must be removed, if they are to fill the places that were designed for them.

This awakening is not confined to our own country, but is extending to all the civilized world, and even shows itself in semi-civilized regions. Such being the present status, it is a favorable time to call the attention of those who are desiring something better for women than has yet been attained to the subject of dress-reform.

When new duties devolve upon us, it is wise to prepare ourselves for their performance. As the sphere of women enlarges, more and more is required of them; and they should therefore throw off all customs that tend to cramp them in any direction, and should endeavor to retain only such as liberate and enlarge their powers, and tend to invigorate both mind and body. In this way alone can they prepare themselves for greater usefulness.

In order to justify ourselves for endeavoring to change the present modes of dress, it is necessary to show that those now in vogue do not answer the reasonable requirements for which clothing was originally designed, and that, instead of being a useful servant wisely fulfilling the purposes of its existence, our dress has become a terrible tyrant, subjecting the human body to its inconvenient, unsightly, and even tormenting control, and bringing into subjection, also, the noble faculties of the mind. By the engrossment of these faculties with the invention of an almost endless variety of unhealthy styles, so much time is necessarily devoted to dress that little or none is left for the higher and better purposes of mental culture. Ever since our first parents clothed themselves with fig-leaves in the garden of Eden, dress has been growing more and more complicated, as the centuries have rolled on, until now it absorbs the attention of many to the exclusion of all nobler thoughts and pursuits.

Its earliest use was for a covering, that our nakedness might not appear; but the climate of a large portion of the globe makes it necessary, in order to protect the body from the inclemencies of the weather and preserve its temperature sufficiently high to prevent the congestions and inflammations that are so dangerous to health and even life.

Let us consider what are the legitimate requirements of clothing, since it appears absolutely indispensable over a large part of the globe. First of all, it should be of such material as will protect the body from the too heating rays of the sun in warm climates, and induce so high a temperature in colder regions that the body will not suffer from chill. In the second place, it should be of such material that its weight will not be an incumbrance, or cause fatigue during exercise. In the third place, it should be so fashioned that its weight will rest mostly upon the shoulders, and not bear too heavily upon the abdominal muscles, as, otherwise, it will lead to displacement and subsequent disease of the internal organs. In the fourth place, it should not press too closely upon any part of the body, lest it obstruct the circulation of the blood, and cause serious disturbances in the whole physical economy. When any thing impedes the current of the blood and prevents its proper aeration and purification, this fluid, instead of being fitted to supply the waste of our bodies, becomes an active agent in producing disease; and the effete matter retained in it is carried to every part of the body, poisoning the very sources of life. In the fifth place, it should be fashioned in such a manner as to furnish the least possible obstruction to locomotion, and indeed to all motion, so that we may be able to walk and work with nearly the same ease as if divested of all covering.

We shall see how poorly these requirements have been fulfilled in the dress worn by women.

The clothing of men, in all Christian countries, has for a long time subserved the legitimate uses for which it was designed. Each part is fitted to the body so as to keep the temperature equable. Its weight is borne on the shoulders; and while it is loose enough to give free circulation, it is yet not loose enough to lessen its protecting power. The dress hats of gentlemen form the most prominent exception to the adaptation of their clothing to proper uses; but those are now little worn, except in dress circles. The covering of men's feet is admirably adapted to their protection from cold and damp, — two great sources of disease. The soles of their boots are broad enough to allow the foot to expand, as Nature designed it should, when pressed upon by the weight of the body; and the toes are wide enough to allow them to rest upon the sole separately, producing the elastic rebound which enables one to walk without fatigue. That there are men foolish enough to cramp their feet in narrow boots, we are aware; but these are a very small minority, and are not the leading ones who are copied by the masses.

The nicely fitting pantaloons, that permit such freedom in the movement of the lower limbs; the snug vests, that preserve a uniform temperature of the chest; and the little sack-coat that, while finishing the toilet, so little inconveniences the wearer; and the over-coat, so easily removed when the temperature of the place renders it unnecessary, — these are all beautifully adapted to their legitimate uses.

It is true that fashion at times renders each of these garments less useful and convenient, as when dandies appear with pantaloons so tight as scarcely to permit bending the knees, or with vests open nearly to the waist that they may display their faultless linen; but these freaks of fashion are of short duration, and the good sense of the masses does not adopt such extremes.

But how has it been with the clothing of women? Has that been more and more conformable to its proper uses? Would that we could say yes. Instead of this being the case, it would almost seem that the ingenuity of the sex had been exercised to find shapes that would most effectually subvert the designs of Nature. The feet have been covered with boots which are wholly inadequate to furnish protection from cold and damp, while they are so shaped as to compress the foot into the narrowest compass, and to crowd the toes upon each other within the narrow tip. This prevents the action of the muscles of the foot in walking, and throws the whole labor upon the muscles of the leg, thus disabling our women from healthful exercise to such a degree that not one in twenty can walk three miles without complete exhaustion.

The Chinese shock our moral sense when they deform the feet of their women by merciless compression in infancy; but we at the same time tolerate — nay, encourage — ours in wearing such covering as lays the foundation for consequences more fatal than theirs. The high heels which have been so fashionable, but which are now, happily, less used, are one of the most fruitful sources of disease. They not only cause contractions of the muscles of the leg, so great in some instances as to make a surgical separation of them necessary, but by raising the heel they bring the weight of the body upon the toes, and thus induce the corns and bunions that alone suffice to make locomotion very painful. Moreover, by inclining the body forward, they throw the uterus out of its normal position, and oblige the ligaments that are designed to steady it to remain constantly in action, in order to restore it to its proper place. These muscles kept continually on the stretch soon lose their contractile power; and then the uterus, thrown out of place by the unnatural pose of the body, remains in this abnormal position, and often becomes adherent to the adjacent parts. When this is the case, a most serious disease is entailed upon the sufferer.

The compression of the calf of the leg by tight ligatures, intended to keep the hose in place, is very injurious, for it often causes distended veins, and checks the natural flow of blood in all the vessels of the leg. We find cramps as the result of this in some cases, numbness in others, and coldness in a great many.

The closed drawers that are worn by most women at the present time are extremely unhealthy, inducing a train of evils which cannot be spoken of here, but which seriously deteriorate the health.

The corsets that encase the body in a prison barred with whalebone and steel are often so closely applied that the action of the muscles within is rendered almost null. This stricture about the waist, by which the liver is so pressed upon that its proper action is greatly obstructed, compresses at the same time the large blood-vessels of the trunk in such a manner as to seriously check the flow of the vital current within. In consequence of this, all the functions of the body are carried on with constantly diminishing force, until the health is completely destroyed and an invalid life makes it impossible longer to endure the pressure of the agent that has wrought such fearful changes in the formerly healthy body.

The evil just spoken of is not always so great as here depicted: it is proportioned to the amount of compression, and the strength of the frame subjected to it. The less the compression, the less the evil; and the more vigorous the body, the better able it is to resist the influence, and to carry on its work in spite of the obstacles that oppose it.

Such consequences as we have mentioned, one might think would be sufficiently alarming to banish from intelligent society the health-destroying corset. But no! The Juggernaut of fashion demands the sacrifice, and its victims must fall down and be crushed by its senseless power.

Next come the skirts, which hang upon the weakened muscles of the abdomen. These garments are often many in number, and at the present time are generally weighted with heavy trimmings reaching to the knee or hips. All this burdensome material is fastened tightly about the waist to prevent dragging; while the skirt is either so long as to obstruct the movement of the feet in walking, or, still worse, it trails upon the dirty sidewalks, gathering up the refuse of the streets, and disgusting those whose sense of neatness makes them shudder to think of the condition of a nice dress after a public promenade.

These long dresses, heavily trimmed, not only entail the evils mentioned, but by their weight drag down the contents of the abdomen, and produce the many diseases peculiar to women, which are the *opprobrium medicale* of the present day. Then comes the over-skirt, which is looped up on the back and sustained there by "bishops" of greater or less weight and density. The mass thus formed heats the spine, prevents the wearer from resting comfortably on chair or seat, and fatigues the back by an unnatural position, as well as by the weight thus heaped upon it. Could any thing more unsightly be invented? Or could one imagine that any lady, who naturally desires to look well and to be prepossessing in her appearance, would willingly array herself in such a costume?

The present short walking-dresses are less objectionable than most that have been worn for a long time; but, in order to have them conform to the proper standard, the over-skirt should be dispensed with, and the length curtailed so that they would just touch the instep, and be of the same length all round. Some simple trimming might be used without impairing their usefulness. The waist, too, should be so loose as to allow the full expansion of the chest with every inspiration.

We had hoped that this short walking-dress, so comfortable and so generally liked, might retain its place in the wardrobe of women; but to our regret and mortification we see it gradually abandoned by almost all, and a demi-train substituted, which outrages all sense of neatness by trailing along the dirty sidewalks. Or, if the wearer would lift it from the ground, she is obliged to swoop it up most ungracefully, or to clutch it still more awkwardly with both hands, thus throwing out the elbows, and reminding one, by the figure she makes, of a turkey displaying his plumage.

The evils arising from tight dressing are too

numerous to be mentioned here, but they are alone sufficient to destroy the health of the most robust person; and even when the pressure thus occasioned is only so little that it is regarded as almost nothing by ladies generally, it is sufficient to lower the standard of health to a considerable degree.

No dress should be so small as to require the least possible effort to fasten it. It should be closed by merely bringing the edges together, without contraction of the chest; and, when closed, the chest should be as free to expand as if nothing covered it. With such garments, the necessity of support from the shoulders will be apparent.

When any injurious garment is first worn, Nature remonstrates, and pain or inconvenience is felt; but if we neglect these monitions, and continue its use, the warning grows less and less loud, until, as it were, discouraged by our wilful neglect of her cautions, Nature ceases to remonstrate. But, though the sufferings first felt are now unnoticed, the penalty is sure to be inflicted, and we pay dearly for our disobedience in impaired health, weakened digestion, poor circulation, diseased liver, restless nights, and the whole host of sufferings that follow in the train of outraged Nature.

I have already made it apparent, I trust, to any one at all acquainted with physiology, that the present style of woman's attire is subversive of the uses which dress should serve, and that a radical change must be made before it can be adapted to health and comfort.

It is desirable that the dress of women should be pleasing to the eye as well as convenient for the uses for which it is designed. The element of beauty is everywhere visible in the creation of God; and the love of it is deeply implanted in our natures, so that "a thing of beauty is a joy for ever." We should not therefore despise the charms that dress can give, nor neglect the adorning of our persons; but we should also remember that health and comfort are not to be sacrificed to beauty, nor our families deprived of the necessaries of life that we may shine in beautiful garments.

Let us remember that the most beautiful costume embraces the idea of use, and of adaptation to the ends that should be sought in all clothing; namely, the sustaining a proper temperature of the body, the lightness necessary to allow easy exercise, and the weight mostly resting on the shoulders. The dress should not fit too closely, lest it may disturb circulation; nor be made so voluminous as greatly to hinder motion, or to make it fatiguing.

There is another point, concerning the dresses of infants, upon which I desire to speak; and I wish I could speak loud enough for every mother in the world to hear. But, as I cannot do this, I will ask you all to aid in extending the word, until, with united power, we may be able to induce all mothers who care more for the health and comfort of their offspring than they do for the behests of fashion to adopt a better dress for their children than is at present worn. Such a dress, being often seen, may in time become fashionable, and then those whose only guide in preparing the wardrobe of the coming child is the reigning style will be led into better modes, so that more convenient and comfortable garments will be made.

The special evil of which I speak is the long skirts, dresses, and cloaks, which are now the fashion for babies. I feel the deepest commiseration for a delicate child that has hung upon its tender body a flannel skirt a yard long, and over that a cotton skirt equally long, and over that a dress to cover both, often weighted with heavy embroidery, and, if the child is carried out, a double cloak longer than all, so that the skirts reach nearly to the floor as the infant is borne on the nurse's arm. The longer the clothes, the more aristocratic the baby, would seem to be the idea of the mother! Think of all this weight attached around the waist of the child, and hanging over the little feet, pressing down the toes, and even forcing the feet out of their natural position! How much of deformity and suffering this fashion produces, none can tell; but that it is a great discomfort to the baby, every thinking mother must perceive.

High necks and long sleeves are now fashionable for babies; but how soon they may be laid aside for low necks and short sleeves cannot be foreseen. That will depend on the enlightenment of women. To expose the delicate chest and arms of a young child in our cold, changeable climate, is often to bring on pneumonia, and greatly to lessen the chances of life. And, should life be spared, there will be sleepless nights and anxious days for the mother, as well as great suffering for the child.

All modes of dress that injure the human body, or make the wearer uncomfortable, are strictly within the province of the doctor; and he should never lose an opportunity to benefit his patients by teaching them the evils to be avoided by a sensible reform in dress. The protest of one physician may do much; but what an incalculable amount of good could be done if the whole profession, as with one voice, would unite in decrying all the forms of dress which torture mankind and bring on the innumerable diseases that shorten life and render it miserable! I speak to you as mothers and sisters who desire to know the best ways to make life healthy and happy for yourselves and for those you love.

There is another evil demanding our earnest consideration, and it is one of the growing evils of the day. I mean the immense labor bestowed on all the garments, and extending to every article that is worn, so that those whose circumstances demand economy must give a large portion of their time to the making and embellishing of their wardrobes. By exhausting strength in too long-continued labor, they deprive themselves of sleep, "tired Nature's sweet restorer," and have no time for intellectual pursuits. Is not the life more than meat, and the body more than raiment? And shall we neglect the soul and intellect God has given us, that we may adorn the perishing body?

Our only hope for the redemption of woman from the thraldom of dress lies in the belief that her hitherto limited sphere of activities has been so insufficient for her intellectual occupations that she has been forced to expend her thoughts in decorating her person, instead of in enlarging her mind. Had she been led to use her executive powers in organizing benevolent enterprises and carrying them out, or in moulding the characters of her children by sharing their higher pursuits, she would not only have impressed herself forcibly upon the institutions of the country, but her mind and heart would have been filled with more ennobling and satisfying enjoyments, and thus the persevering efforts now made to frivolous ends would have been turned into channels of usefulness.

It is, however, better that the feminine intellect should have been actively employed in inventing new forms of dress and embellishment, than that it should have lain dormant, and been reduced to almost complete inanition for want of any activity. By this exercise of its powers, it has been in a measure strengthened and prepared for the important labors which will soon be required of it.

The day is not far distant when woman is to take part in all which concerns humanity; and the added responsibility that such freedom must bring should stimulate her to be worthy of the blessings to be conferred, which, when they come, will place her where her influence will be as extensive as her abilities and contributions to the general good deserve.

If she is to fulfil the high trusts that shall be given her, she must emancipate herself from the engrossments of fashion, must be clothed in garments that will contribute to her comfort, and must cast aside those that destroy her health, cripple her energies, and take all her time and means for their manufacture. She must seek first the liberal education that has so long been considered necessary for her brothers, in order that they may be prepared for the varied duties that are required of them. When the leading women of the age, and those blessed with wealth and high position, come to see that a cultivated mind in a healthy body is more to be desired, and better calculated to lead to honor and esteem, than the most costly or elaborate clothing, women will turn their attention to these higher objects, and will then make it easy for others less favored to follow in the same pathway. A great responsibility is resting upon women who are blessed with the wealth and station that carry so much influence with them. They could easily change the fashions of dress so as to remove the objections to present modes, and by so doing they would contribute greatly to the health and happiness of the wearers.

The lavish expenditure in dress, so common at the present time, is a matter of serious concern to those who reflect much upon its tendencies. Society, by denying to women the propriety of earning money, or of entering into any business that will make them self-supporting, fixes the badge of poverty upon all who attempt to provide in this manner for their own or their families' wants. Thus the burden of mortified pride is added to the exhausting labor of self-support, which is also rendered heavier for women than for men by the inferior wages the former receive, and by the necessarily higher cost of their wardrobe when they procure it made for themselves, as men procure theirs. In consequence of this expense, women seek to eke out their small incomes by sewing their own clothes; and, when engaged in business, this must be done after the regular task of the day is finished. Such wearying occupation often keeps them at work till the small hours of the night, and thus deprives them of the rest which is needful to refresh their tired bodies, and to render them fit for the labor of the coming day. We need not wonder that many women break down under these accumulated burdens, especially when we consider that they have to do all this in clothing not fitted to preserve health, but rather calculated to fetter their powers, and to make work and motion a painful effort. Headaches and indigestions must result from the constant application of eyes, mind, and muscles to this most sedentary of all employments; and the persons so occupied become depressed in spirits, unacquainted with the activities of the world, and little fitted to bear their part in those conversations and amusements which should make the family the centre of intellectual and affectional enjoyments, and which alone can retain husbands and brothers in the pure and tranquillizing atmosphere of a happy and cultivated home.

We are a republican nation, at least in form, and have no distinct classes where the lines are so tightly drawn that citizens cannot pass from one to the other. In accord with the genius of our institutions, all desire to attain to the highest places; and consequently an elevating impulse is given, which is calculated to foster enterprise and thrift, and to ennoble the people by the stimulus of a possibility of reaching places of honor and profit, even from the lowest points. This is one of the greatest blessings that a republican government confers upon its people. We should therefore, as good citizens and as Christian women, do all we can to foster this self-respect in those less favored than ourselves, and should never think that their depression will elevate us.

I know it will be said that the wealthy have a perfect right to indulge in all the luxuries that they may choose, and that they help the poorer classes by distributing money amongst them, when they hire them to make their elaborate garments. But let us look carefully at this matter, and see if it will bear the test of close examination. Is it a benefit to the poor sempstress to give her more sewing, when at the same time we oblige her, by our example, to spend all she gets for it in adorning her own dresses, that she may appear respectably in the presence of the elegantly clothed ladies who patronize her? Has any one a right to destroy the beautiful body God has given, or even to injure its wonderful mechanism and to throw it out of balance, so that it can perform its intended work only with great pain and suffering? Has any one a right to tempt others to do wrong, or by example to lead them on to destroy their vigor and usefulness by unhealthful modes of dress, or by the overwork needed to embellish them? Did not the great Apostle Paul teach us our duty in these respects, when he said, "If meat make my brother to offend, I will eat no flesh while the world standeth"? Have not all of us duties to society and to our fellow-beings that should never be lost sight of? And have we not still higher duties to our Maker, which require us to preserve the health of our bodies, that we may be able to perform the work He intended for us? And, finally, have we not a duty to our country, to check, as far as we can, the growing evils of extravagance that are now undermining the very foundations of our social life, and threatening to demoralize it?

There is still another class of women who are seriously injured by the elaborate style of clothing now worn by all classes, and this is the middle class, who live in handsome, well-furnished residences, and make a fine appearance at church and on the street, and who yet cannot afford to hire their dressmaking done. Not recognizing the truth that all useful labor is honorable, and desiring to appear more wealthy than they really are, they are led by false pride to conceal the fact that they are their own dressmakers.

The burden of making these over-trimmed dresses falls heavily upon them, and, by keeping them in the house plying the needle, it deprives them of that daily out-of-door exercise which is so necessary to vigorous health. Thus all the time left from the cares of home is spent in the excessive ornamentation demanded by the tyranny of fashion, and none is found for reading or intellectual pursuits of any sort.

Nor are these the only evils arising from the extravagant modes of dress, and the extravagant style of living which accompanies them; for the husband or father who loves his family is unwilling to deny them the money necessary to purchase these elegancies, and he often goes beyond his means that his family may appear as well as his neighbor's. This leads him to incur obligations which he cannot meet, and financial embarrassment and ruin stare him in the face. If he is in a place of trust, he is tempted to borrow, as he leniently calls it, from the funds that have been placed in his hands, thinking that he can soon return the sum, and that no one will be the wiser or be injured by what he does. But at last, after many shifts, he can no longer conceal the deficit; and then he is ruined in purse and character, thrust out of his place, and sometimes brought to self-destruction by the desperation that follows his exposure!

Is not society accountable in a great measure for these and similar breaches of trust in private citizens and public servants? And who but women control the customs of society, and make them either prudent, wise, and moral, or extravagant, foolish, and immoral? I appeal to the moral sense of the ladies present, and I ask them if they are willing, by their example and influence, longer to countenance a mode of dress which is so little fitted to answer the reasonable demands that should be made upon it, and so destructive of health and of morals?

If we have convinced you that the serious charges brought against the dress of the present day are well founded, you will surely be unwilling longer to participate in its follies, not to say in its crimes against the peace and welfare of society.

What, then, shall be done to inaugurate a true reform in this important direction?

To answer this may require wiser heads than ours; but the first step is taken when women are convinced that there is need of reform. After that, clear heads and tender consciences will address themselves to the task, and will soon find ways to accomplish it. Combination and organization are required to assist in the work, and numerical strength is needed to overcome long-established customs. What would be martyrdom for a few to attempt would be easy for masses to accomplish. If five hundred earnest, intelligent women should band themselves together, and agree to discard as soon as possible all garments that prove injurious to health, and should then set their inventive faculties to work to produce a simple and beautiful style of apparel that might be free from the objections brought against our present modes, — a style which should have the great merit of pleasing the artistic sense, and becoming the wearer, and in which age, condition of life, and personal peculiarities would be so considered as to make each dress appropriate to its owner, and expressive of her character, instead of being a mere duplicate of some other garment, without regard to personal fitness, — could this be done, the needed work of dress-reform would be half accomplished. Let us not attempt to imitate the fashions of the Old World, which are unsuited to our republican nation, and not in accord with our institutions. We are a young and vigorous people, and should no more attempt to copy the dress and style of living of the European nations than we do their laws and institutions. Let us be the inventors of our own fashions, and let them conform to the character of our institutions in their simplicity and adaptation to our peculiar wants, and then they will become the exponent of our own nationality.

LECTURE IV.

BY ARVILLA B. HAYNES, M.D.

LADIES, — When I was invited to take part in these lectures on Dress-Reform, I consented to do so, not because I thought I was qualified above others to speak or teach on this subject, but because I felt a deep interest in what was to be brought before you.

I consider the theme one of great importance, — so great, indeed, that it cannot be overestimated. When we see disease the rule, and health the exception, it seems fitting for women to pause and inquire the cause of this unnatural state of things. And the answer comes back to us from every side, "There is a perversion of the natural functions, and a disregard of hygienic laws."

In the brief time allotted to a single lecture, it would be impossible to exhaust a subject of so much interest, or one so fruitful of good and ill to mankind. As it has been my privilege to observe from the standpoint of a physician, I shall speak from the same, hoping by so doing to speak with greater authority. And my endeavor will be to present to you the practical side of this question, leaving the artistic and æsthetic for other hands. If I repeat any thing that has been said by those who have preceded me, I hope you will consider the statement to be of so much importance that it insists upon arresting your attention.

I propose to speak on the influence of external conditions on the human body.

The conditions that demand our attention in connection with the subject before us are mechanical pressure, and sudden alternations of temperature arising from the application of cold and dampness to the surface of the body. Both of these conditions are greatly affected by our artificial covering, — the dress.

As we approach this temple of nature, the human body, examine its structure and observe its perfect adaptation to uses, we see much that excites our wonder and admiration. Looking at the lowest forms of animal life, we find they are made up of an aggregation of cells, every part like every other part, and all homogeneous in character. As we rise a little in the scale, there is a differentiation of parts: organs are developed, at first rudimentary. A little higher still, these organs are more fully developed, and others are added. And so on, until we pass through the different classes, and arrive at the vertebrate animals and man.

In these highest organisms, where work is to be done, there is a division of the labor, and organs and systems are set apart to perform certain functions. In studying this complex structure, we must first understand its anatomy, or the normal relation of one part to another, before we can understand deformities, or a departure from the normal relation. We must also understand its physiology, or the functions of the several systems or organs, before we can understand any perversion of these functions.

So you will allow me to examine a little the body we would properly clothe, and see the relation of one part to another, also the functions these several organs and systems are called upon to perform. By so doing we shall better understand the influence of the external conditions furnished by dress.

We see the human body as a symmetrical whole. It has a bony framework or skeleton, that gives form and outline to the body. This is clothed with muscles, that are traversed by a system of glands, and permeated by blood-vessels and nerves. Over all is placed a covering, the integument or skin.

Within, we find three great cavities, — the cranial cavity, the cavity of the chest, and the abdominal cavity. Within the cavity of the cranium is lodged that great nervous centre, the brain; and intimately connected with this is the spinal cord, enclosed in a bony canal. From these two nervous centres proceed nerves of sensation and of voluntary motion, which serve as channels of communication to all parts of the body.

The cavity of the chest is formed principally by the ribs, attached to the vertebræ posteriorly, and to the sternum anteriorly, by cartilage. Its walls are more or less flexible. Within the chest the heart and lungs are located.

Below the chest we have the abdominal cavity, with muscular walls. It contains the liver on the right, on the left the spleen, the stomach somewhat to the left, and the alimentary canal arranged in convolutions. Below, in the pelvis, are found the organs of generation.

Each organ contained in these several cavities has its own peculiar work to perform; and this brings us to a consideration of the various systems.

The digestive system lies at the foundation of all the organic functions; for on this organized beings depend for their growth, development, and maintenance during life. After a nutrient fluid has been elaborated by the digestive organs from the alimentary substances they receive, it must be conveyed to all parts of the body to be assimilated; hence the circulating system. This nutrient fluid must be maintained in a state of purity, and we have excreting organs. The kidneys belong to the excreting organs; and the function of the skin is correlated to that of the kidneys. The respiratory system is of importance in maintaining the blood in a state of purity, as it performs the double office of removing carbonic acid and of introducing oxygen. All these are separate and distinct functions, yet they are mutually dependent on one another; and on their uniform and harmonious operation the life of the individual depends.

In the normal condition, or in a state of health, these functions go on without consciousness; that is, they are involuntary. The heart pulsates with the same regularity, asleep or awake; respiration, also, is carried on in a tranquil and uniform manner. The kidneys fulfil their office of excretion; and the skin is at all times eliminating the substances that would be deleterious if allowed to remain in the system. The stomach, likewise, performs its part of the digestive process, without entering any protest through the nervous system.

The functions that are of primary importance to us in considering the influence of external conditions are the circulation and the respiration; and of these I wish to speak more fully. They also hold an important place among the organic functions.

The circulating system consists of the heart, the arteries, capillaries, and veins, and the fluid contained therein, — the blood. Of this system the heart is the central organ; and it is a muscle of great strength in proportion to its size. The arteries are hollow tubes, somewhat elastic, and with a contractile power. They are always full. They convey blood from the heart, and begin there as one large vessel; but soon they send off branches that divide and subdivide, till they terminate in numerous minute capillaries, that are intermediate between the arteries and veins. The capillaries are microscopic in size, and form a network in the tissues. The veins begin at the capillaries; and as they go towards the heart they unite, until they terminate at the heart as two large vessels, one bringing the blood from the head and upper extremities, and the other from the trunk and lower extremities. The arteries convey the blood outward from the heart, and are deep-seated; the veins return the blood to the heart, and are both deep-seated and superficial. The veins return the blood of the general circulation to the right auricle of the heart. From this it is forced into the right ventricle, thence into the pulmonary artery, and then it is conveyed to the lungs. From the lungs it is returned by the pulmonary veins to the left auricle of the heart; it then passes into the left ventricle, and from this into the arteries; and is then conveyed over the system, and returned again to the right side of the heart.

This is the general circulation, and it is carried on with great rapidity. The whole amount of blood in the body is estimated as about one-fifth or one-eighth of its weight; so that in a body weighing 120 lbs. we should have about 15 lbs. of blood. The capacity of the chambers of the heart is from $1\frac{1}{2}$ to 2 oz. With the lower estimate, the heart pulsating sixty times per minute, which is the average rate, the whole amount of blood in the system will pass through the heart in about three minutes. The circulation, when unimpeded, is carried on in a regular and uniform manner, every part receiving its normal quantity of blood. The lungs, located upon the right and left sides of the chest, are essentially composed of the blood-vessels, and the numerous and minute divisions of the bronchi that terminate in a cluster of air-cells. They are supplied with nerves and glands, and are all held together by a delicate tissue or membrane. We see the same arrangement of the blood-vessels in the lungs as elsewhere. The pulmonary artery enters the lungs as one large vessel, and divides into numerous minute branches, terminating in capillaries; and the veins begin at the capillaries, as small vessels that unite and return the blood to the left auricle of the heart. The circulation of the blood through the lungs is termed the lesser circulation; but it is a very important part of the economy of the system. The arrangement of the blood-vessels in the lungs serves admirably for the re-creation and purification of the blood. The minute capillaries form a network around the air-cells, and the blood is separated from the air in the cells by the most delicate of tissues, which allows only gases to pass through it. Here the exchange is made: the blood takes oxygen from the respired air, and gives up the carbon which it has received from waste material, and which acts as a poison when it remains in the system.

Respiration is one of the most important of the organic functions; and it is only by the constant and uniform flow of blood through the lungs, — and it passes through the lungs with the same rapidity that it passes through the heart, — and the no less constant and regular act of respiration, that the blood is kept in a condition to serve the purpose of nutrition.

Let us now look at the influence of mechanical pressure on these functions, which are performed in such a regular and uniform manner by a structure so complicated and delicate. In the arrangement of the organs in the cavities of the body there are no empty spaces. Every organ is in close relation to some other part or organ; and when one is pressed out of its normal position it must encroach on the space allotted to another. The chest-walls are more or less flexible; and when mechanical pressure is made around the lower portion of the chest, and over the free or floating ribs, it lessens materially the capacity of the cavity of the chest, and interferes very essentially with the full and free expansion of the lungs.

When the air-cells of the lungs are not filled with air at every inspiration, the blood is imperfectly aerated. The amount of oxygen supplied by the respired air is not in proportion to the amount of carbon to be eliminated. Consequently the blood remains more or less carbonized, and is unfit for the purpose of nutrition. This condition of the blood reacts on the nervous system, and through it on all the organic functions. The free action of the heart is impeded, also the regular contractions of the diaphragm, — that great muscle by which tranquil respiration is performed. The liver is displaced, and encroaches upon the space of the other abdominal organs. The free movement of the stomach is impeded, if active digestion is going on in that organ.

When pressure is made over this region, there cannot be natural motion in any part of the body. As soon as vigorous exercise is engaged in, every part of the system calls for oxygen. In order to supply it, the lungs take on increased action : respiration is quickened. Instead of breathing sixteen times per minute, the normal number, the respiratory effort is increased to twenty per minute ; yet at this rapid rate the lungs are unable to meet the demands made upon them, and fatigue soon follows. All vital acts are peculiarly destructive of their agents.

The corset, as now manufactured and worn, is loosely hooked around the waist. Owing to its own weight and to that of the clothing buttoned over it, it drops down till it rests upon the hips. This arrangement does not remove the pressure caused by the dragging down of skirts at the waist: it only changes it from one point to another, and the result is equally injurious. When the clothing is worn in this way, pressure is made over the abdomen, the convolutions of the intestines are crowded together, and the weight of all the contents of the abdomen is thrown, more or less, upon the organs within the pelvis.

The steel spring in the front of the corset is used as a support for the body. It presses upon the stomach, causing tenderness of the great *solar plexus* of the sympathetic nerves that lie posterior to the stomach. It weakens the abdominal muscles, and destroys in a measure the true vertical bearing of the body.

When this vertical bearing of the body is maintained, every part above rests upon that below. The head rests upon the upper part of the vertebral column, the weight of the trunk upon the hips; and the same plan is carried out through the lower extremities to the arch of the foot. When the body is in this position, the vertebral column has two curves, — a lesser curve above, that gives increased capacity to the chest, and a greater one below. Then the abdominal muscles are tense, and the weight of the contents of the abdomen is thrown upon the pubic portion of the pelvis. But when these muscles are weakened and relaxed, and the greater and lower curve in the spinal column is impaired, owing to pressure from above, the weight of the contents of the abdomen is thrown into the pelvic cavity, causing displacement and prolapsis of the organs situated there.

Since strings have been discarded, and firm hooks and eyes used to fasten the corset, there may have been a decrease in chest diseases, but there has been a corresponding increase in uterine diseases. Some of the mechanical supports that have been invented for uterine displacements are adjusted with the design of restoring the natural curve in the lower portion of the vertebral column, thus giving the abdominal muscles their true lifting power, and throwing the weight of the abdominal viscera upon the pubic bones of the pelvis, where it belongs.

When questioned, ladies rarely admit that

they wear their clothing tight. The hand can be readily passed under the bands, when the diaphragm is relaxed and the air is expelled from the lungs, and their garments are therefore considered loose and comfortable. They do appear to be so; but this is apparent rather than real. If the chest is subjected to pressure for a considerable length of time, it adapts itself to that condition; and we can go on increasing the pressure gradually, until we have contracted chest-walls and displacement of the abdominal organs. Such is the effect of habit on the system.

When the habit is injurious, the changes it effects may be slow and imperceptible, but they will break out ultimately in disease. For, although there is a certain amount of tolerance in the system, no natural law can be disregarded from day to day without bringing, sooner or later, a certain retribution; and the length of time before it appears will be just in proportion to the nature of the abuse and the amount of vital force that there is to resist it.

Let us now try the opposite experiment, and begin to increase the size of the bands, and to allow a little more room for the movements of the vital organs. If we continue to do this from time to time, till the bands have been lengthened three or four inches, at the end of a year we shall find that they are about as tight as when we began to enlarge them. But in this case the tendency will have been towards health. The chest-walls have expanded, and respiration has been more perfectly performed. The diaphragm discharges its natural function; the circulation is unimpeded; and there is greater freedom in all the movements of the body.

Mechanical pressure at any point retards the onward flow of the blood through the veins to the heart. The veins are superficial, or near the surface; and pressure around the limbs at any point will cause a passive congestion of the vessels below that point. This can be readily demonstrated. If you compress the veins of the wrist or arm, in a few minutes the veins of the hand and arm will be swollen. The blood cannot return to the heart. The same takes place if there is pressure at any point around the lower extremities, or on any of the large veins.

One of the important conditions to be maintained in the adjustment of our clothing is a uniform temperature over the surface of the body, without pressure and with the least weight. In our climate, flannel or woollen goods, as a general rule, should be worn next to the skin over the whole body, from the neck to the wrists and ankles. If there is any idiosyncrasy which prevents this material from being thus worn, it should be used as the second covering.

All the clothing should be supported from the shoulder. The corset should be discarded; but if it must be retained as an indispensable article of dress, as it is now considered, it should be made without whalebone or steel springs, and should be held up by a band over the shoulder. All the under-clothing external to this should either be attached to it, or so arranged that the weight may rest on the shoulder. This may be managed by means of suspenders, or by a waist fitted to the form. The less the weight, the better, provided the necessary warmth is secured.

The length of the bands around the waist should be sufficient to allow the utmost freedom to all the movements. Nothing ought to interfere with the action of the abdominal muscles and the diaphragm; and the greatest chest capacity should be secured, in order to enable the lungs to perform properly the function of respiration.

The skirts should be short enough to clear the pavement, and to prevent their lower edges from becoming damp. They should also allow freedom to the feet and limbs in that most healthful of all out-of-door exercise, — walking. No elastic bands should encircle the limbs at any point, as they retard circulation by compressing the blood-vessels. The stockings may be upheld by elastic bands attached at the waist to that portion of the clothing which has its support from the shoulder.

When the clothing is arranged in this way, all

the weight hanging from the shoulder and no pressure at any point, there is freedom of motion in every part. The organs are all in their true relation to one another, and their functions go on unimpeded.

When the temperature is such as to require extra clothing or wraps for the chest and upper extremities, the lower extremities also should receive attention. In the inclement season, when we are liable to sudden alternations of temperature, if the thermometer drops down to zero or near that point, and we go from furnace-heated houses into the open air, we put on cloaks or shawls, furs, and wraps of various kinds; and encase our hands, not only in gloves or mittens, but in muffs. This is all right, and should be done; but it is not sufficient. To the lower extremities we should also add leggins, and a pair of over-drawers made either of ladies' cloth or flannel; and, in wet weather, overshoes.

When one part of the body is over-heated, and another part exposed, the nerves of the exposed part are rendered more sensitive to receive impressions.

In treating of the influence of alternations of temperature which arise from the application of cold to the surface of the body, I shall use the word *cold* as meaning the absence of heat or caloric. Heat and light act externally as stimulants, and are among the conditions essential to life and health. The normal temperature of the body internally is one hundred degrees; on the surface, it is ninety-eight; and the vital functions cannot be carried on if the temperature is lowered in a considerable degree for any length of time.

Cold is a sedative, and when applied to the surface of the body it lowers the vital powers. It acts on the circulation by contracting the blood-vessels; and thus the blood is driven within from the exposed region. If one part is deprived of its normal quantity of blood, another part must have more than its normal quantity, consequently there must be congestion of some of the internal organs. This is what takes place when the extremities are too thinly clad to maintain an equal temperature over the surface. The lungs and the uterine organs are very liable to congestions from this cause, and this is particularly true in regard to girls at the age of puberty. At that period, the vital powers have been developing and perfecting the system, which is then very susceptible of external influences. Exposure to cold at this age often leads to derangements that become chronic, impairing the general health, and causing a vast amount of suffering, while in many cases they establish right conditions for the development of disease in after life. Who among us cannot trace sad results to only a cold?

A proper clothing of the extremities is one of the best preventives; and we may have congestion of any of the internal organs from a failure to do this.

When there is exposure to sudden changes of temperature, without sufficient clothing for protection, the impression on the nerves and on the circulation is often the exciting cause of acute disease. If we look over our medical works as authorities, we find a large number of diseases that are referable to this cause. Who has not observed the prevalence of coughs and colds, as soon as there is a change in the seasons, and summer passes into autumn? This is because there is not a corresponding change in the clothing. The function of the skin as an eliminating organ is checked from these sudden alternations; and substances that should be removed remain in the system. When we remember that from one to three pounds of fluid pass off through the pores of the skin during every twenty-four hours, we see how important it is that the surface of the body should be kept at a proper and equable temperature for its normal action.

The externals of dress, though they involve a moral question, seem to me of far less consequence than the arrangement of the under-dress, for that involves health. As now generally worn, the under-dress is weakening the present generation of women; and, from the unvarying laws of nature, the effect must be transmitted to future generations. Mothers will confer upon their offspring a lower and lower vitality; and, when we consider the already fearful mortality in infancy and childhood, there is little hope for the future, unless we can have some reform in this direction. And when the offspring is not thus early cut off from mortal life, in many cases tendencies to disease are inherited, which become active sooner or later; and thus life is robbed of usefulness and enjoyment. Instead of being self-maintaining and efficient co-workers with their fellows, such children find the burden of physical disability laid upon them; and they drag out a miserable existence, looking forward to a release from their physical weakness into that greater freedom of life and activity that they hope awaits them.

There is to-day a growing prejudice against medication; and, when disease invades the system, many seek through physical culture the means of restoration to health. The adoption of a hygienic dress would be one of the best preventives of disease; and often some such reform is absolutely necessary before strength can be regained.

To me the future looks hopeful, when women realize the cause of this tendency to disease, when they ask for knowledge of their own organisms, and inquire the way back to Nature. Let them but understand what they seek to know, — give them a knowledge of their own organisms, of the relation of one part to another, and a knowledge of the functions these organs are called upon to perform, — let them understand also the unvarying physical laws, and the certain retribution that follows their perversion, and thus enlightened, with their naturally quick perceptions, and their skill in adapting means to ends, they will soon render the dress of every woman and child conformable to the requirements of health.

Then, there will be harmony throughout the whole human system. Every part will be in its true relation to every other part. All the functions will go on without consciousness. Women will not know they have a nervous system merely from the complaints it makes of abuses, but they will understand its higher offices.

The digestive apparatus will properly prepare the alimentary substances it receives into a nutrient fluid, to be conveyed to all parts of the system for their assimilation. The capacity of the lungs to oxygenize and decarbonize the blood will be equal to the demands made upon them, and the excreting organs will remove all waste and worn-out material from the body. No protest from any part of the system will be transmitted through the nerves of sensation to the seat of consciousness, the brain. There will be harmony, also, in the mental condition. The mind will be clear, all the faculties active, and every part amenable to the will will be quick to do its bidding. The spiritual, when not borne down by the physical, rises to loftier heights; and there is harmony throughout the whole being, in a threefold sense.

Let every woman feel the importance of these things, and let her appreciate the duties and responsibilities that rest upon her. Here is a large field for missionary labor; and every one of my hearers should be the good angel that scatters seeds of truth along her daily pathway. Do not excuse yourself by saying, I have not time or opportunity; but begin here and now. Begin with your child, your friend and neighbor; and remember for your encouragement the promise that "to him that hath shall be given." The time has come for these things; and let us hope the day is not far distant when the injunction to "know thyself" will be heeded by the many, instead of the few. A better humanity must result from awakening in the minds of women a desire for knowledge on matters connected with their physical welfare. When this knowledge is at length gained, every child will receive a transmitted organism that shall enable the good and true aspirations born in his soul to find right conditions for developing and blossoming into Christian grace. His life will bear fruit in Christian work here on earth; and its continuance hereafter will be the consummation of all that has gone before.

LECTURE V.

BY ABBA GOOLD WOOLSON.

LADIES, — In coming before you to close this series of lectures upon the reforms needed in woman's dress, I should be presumptuous indeed, were I to speak in detail of the physical discomfort and disease to which our present style of dress inevitably leads. If the able physicians who have preceded me have not made such truths apparent, in their authoritative and emphatic statements, it would be beyond my power to do so. With no consultation together as to the views they should advance, these several physicians, young and middle-aged, trained in different parts of our country, and some of them in Europe, of varied learning and experience and of different schools, have agreed in their assertions that the dress commonly worn to-day by American women is a prolific source

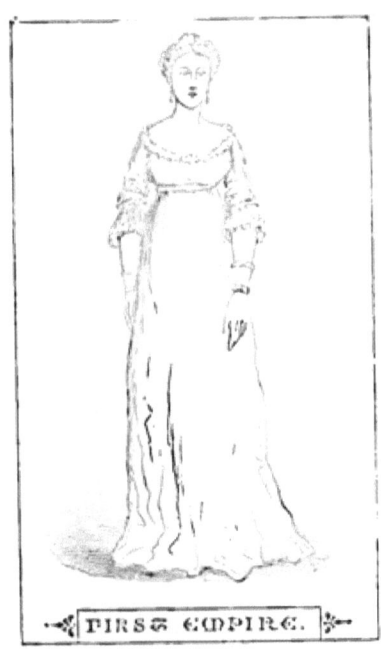

FIRST EMPIRE.

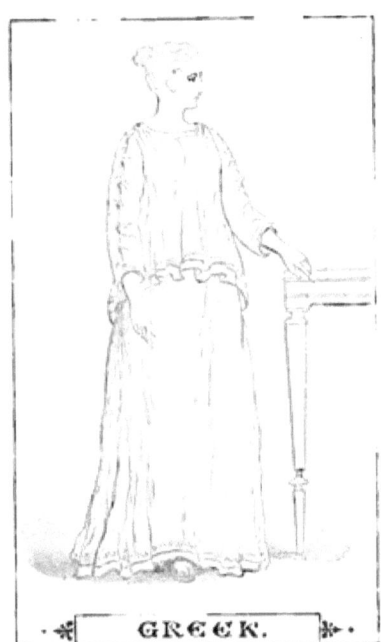

GREEK.

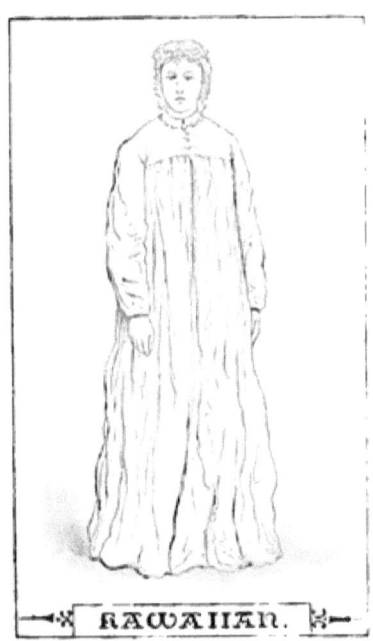

HAWAIIAN.

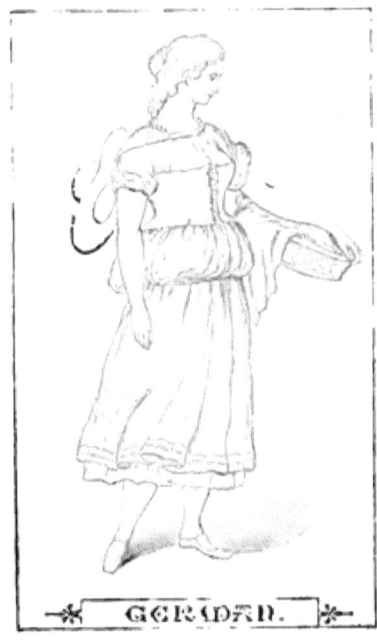

GERMAN.

of bodily weakness and suffering; and that, if adhered to, its tendency must be, not only to enfeeble the powers of women themselves, but seriously to impair the physical strength of the whole nation. No difference of opinion has appeared as to the precise nature of the evils thus engendered, or the measures that should be taken to stay their course.

I may therefore assume that no further argument is needed to demonstrate that the requirements of health and the styles of female attire which custom enjoins are in direct antagonism to each other. But, before passing to the consideration of other phases of the question, not yet touched upon, it may be well to sum up these antagonisms, as they have been presented at length, in a few brief and general statements.

It has been plainly shown that our present dress violates health in three important ways: first, by its compression of vital parts of the body; second, by its great weight, and the faulty suspension of this weight; and, third, by the unequal temperature which it induces.

Thus, Health would say: "If your dress is to be tight, let it be tight anywhere but over the region between the upper, fastened ribs and the hips. If its weight is to be great, let it hang from the solid framework of the shoulders, not from this sensitive central region where there is nothing to support it. If any part is to be overheated, let it be the extremities, and not this. For here lie the vital organs whose unimpeded action is essential to your very life, — the lungs, the heart, the liver, and the stomach. That they may have the fullest opportunity to expand and move, they are covered only with loose flesh and a few movable bones."

But Custom says: "Let your dress be tight nowhere but over this very region between the ribs and the hips. Loosen your clothing over the bone-encased shoulders; from your hips to your feet hang wide-floating draperies; but bind and pinch and tighten over the lower air-cells of the lungs, over the throbbing heart, the active liver, and the expanding stomach. Fortunately there is nothing there, by way of bones, to prevent you from squeezing yourself all you wish; and only by squeezing yourself there can you be made beautiful in my eyes."

She says also: "You are weaker than man in physical strength, from a lack of exercise in youth, and from an in-door life. Carry, then, about yourself four times as much weight as he; multiply your garments; lengthen your skirts; weigh them down with ornament; and gird them all over the shelf of your hips. There they will drag upon stomach and intestines, but I do not concern myself about that."

When Health insists upon an equality of temperature, with a greater amount of clothing over the extremities in order to insure this equal warmth, Custom, as antagonistic as ever, has these orders to give: "Clothe slightly legs and arms; but encompass your body, just where the active internal organs create the most heat, with a torrid zone, an inch or two in width, of twenty thicknesses of material in the form of bindings. Below these, plait, gather, and reduplicate your cloth till it is ten-fold the thickness it is above the belted zone from which the skirts depend. If the nerve-centres that lie beneath, in stomach and spine, become weakened and disordered, it is nothing to me."

Health says also: "Have your dress durable and simple, that you may go abroad readily in all weathers, and be afraid of neither sun, rain, nor wind." But Custom makes it perishable in fabric, and engrossing in the care it demands; and, being also burdensome and tight, it discourages exercise, save of the mildest sort and in the blandest weather.

Such differences as these which have been pointed out are too broad to be reconciled. Who can wonder that we seek to change Custom, and to work a reform in her requirements, since the physical laws with which these conflict must remain for ever inflexible?

In considering the hygienic aspect of this subject, physicians remember not only the daily physical discomfort and suffering of women, but the excessive agonies which child-birth brings upon them, the frequent death which it entails, and the inferior children to which such mothers must inevitably give birth. A leading female physician of Philadelphia is convinced, from her own observation, that there has been an alarming increase of ill-health among women during even the past two years, and that maternity is fast becoming an unnaturally fearful peril. She believes the dress commonly worn to-day to be the cause of all this.

That weakness and disease are not inherent in our sex, as is too commonly supposed, will be plainly apparent, if we remember the strength and vigor possessed by the women of savage tribes, of the toiling peasant classes of Europe, and of the harems of the East. What makes the difference in this respect between them and the ladies of Europe and America? No medical authority who has ever worn the dress of the latter can doubt that the habitual disregard of physical laws which it imposes will alone suffice to account for the existence of all their diseases, new and old. Medical authorities who have never worn it may look far and wide for other causes, but it is because they ignore or undervalue evils which they have never experienced.

We are ready to trace a connection between two facts which Mrs. Leonowens states concerning Siamese women; viz., that they wear only a few ounces of loose silk cloth for covering, and that they are wholly ignorant of the long train of female weaknesses of which we hear so much.

Looking over the world at large, it would appear that, just in proportion as a nation advances in general intelligence and Christian virtue, in just that proportion does the female half of its people delight in dressing so as to defy Nature's laws. It is a curious anomaly, which I will not stop to explain. So long as women remain heathen, they may be servile, ignorant, and frivolous, but they do appear to have some respect for their bodies. The free-flowing outlines of the costumes worn by Greek and Roman maids and matrons were not more beautiful to the eye of the artist, as he pictured them in the sacred processions that wind across their vases and bas-reliefs, than they were conducive to the full development of that body whose strength and beauty their people worshipped with such reverent homage. And could mothers begirt with corsets, laced and panniered after the modes of our time, have given birth to the race of athletic young heroes who strove before their assembled countrymen for the crowns of honor at national games? All the women of the East, as well as those of Siam, drape themselves to-day with light folds of unsewed cloth, and know nothing of our elaborate fastenings and complicated layers of inconveniences. Of the women of the Sandwich Islands, a traveller tells us: "Their loose dress gives grace as well as dignity to their movements, and whoever invented it for them deserves more credit than he has received. It is a little startling at first to see women walking about in what, to our perverted taste, looks like calico or black stuff nightgowns; but the dress grows on you as you become accustomed to it. It lends itself readily to bright ornamentation; it is eminently fit for the climate; and a stately Hawaiian dame, marching through the street in black *holaku,* as the dress is called, with a long necklace, or *le,* of bright scarlet or brilliant yellow flowers, bare and untrammelled feet, and flowing hair, compares very favorably with a high-heeled, wasp-waisted, absurdly bonneted white lady." Barbarous tribes allow still greater ease and freedom in their attire.

But cross the boundaries of any civilized and Christian land, and you behold a race of gasping, nervous, and despairing women, who, with their compressed ribs, torpid lungs, hobbling feet, and bilious stomachs, evidently consider it their first duty to mortify the flesh, and to render themselves and all humanity belonging to them as frail and uncomfortable as possible. If it be true that the New Testament and the Parisian fashion-book do necessarily go hand in hand, we might well hesitate before sending more missionaries abroad to the happy heathen, endeavoring to save their souls while making sure of ruining their bodies.

But no dress of any time or of any land, be it Pagan or Christian, would answer the requirements which we make to-day. Were all the costumes ever devised spread out before us for our choice, it is doubtful if we should find ourselves well served with any. For the present was not comprehended in the past; and our sisters abroad know little of the duties that we must meet or of the ideas which shape our lives.

The world of the past appears to have asked itself only this question concerning woman, "Is she made to work, or to be looked at?" "To work," replied the barbarous races; and half clad, like the rest of her tribe, she then found little hindrance in her clothes. No dress-reform was needed for her. "To be looked at," said the Eastern nations, and they still drape her like a helpless doll. But where active, out-door life is forbidden, a dress suited to dawdling about divanned courts is all that is required. "Both to work, and to be looked at," say the civilized peoples of the West; and here, wrapped in the loose folds of the harem, she strives to labor like her sisters of the forest. If the draperies have been somewhat lengthened and tightened, if the labors have become more multiform, and are carried on mostly in-doors, it makes the matter no better for her. In all these cases, her own claims and her own feelings are as utterly ignored as if she were a senseless stone.

But a new clause is added to these hitherto approved replies. To-day, woman herself, educated, enterprising, ambitious, has something to say in her own behalf. "Yes," she assents, "woman was made to work, to be looked at, but also to enjoy her own life; living not only for others, but for herself, and most helpful when most true to her own needs."

This is the new doctrine which she is preaching to our age. "I exist," she says, "not as wife, not as mother, not as teacher, but, first of all, as woman, with a right to existence for my own sake."

Believing this, she makes a new demand upon her attire. She must still work in it, she must still look beautiful in it, but she must also be strong and comfortable and happy in it. It is in this requirement which she makes of her present dress that it fails her the most. She does manage to accomplish a deal of earnest work in it, though much less than she is capable of doing. The generations which she must please think she looks beautiful in it, since their eyes have become accustomed to its ugliness; but she finds herself borne down by its weight, breathless from its compressions, and weary with buffeting its opposing folds.

Of all nations of the earth, we suffer the most from the cruel tyrannies of dress. None need a serviceable costume so much as we, and none have one so bad. Indeed, American ladies are known abroad for two distinguishing traits (besides, possibly, their beauty and self-reliance), and these are their ill-health and their extravagant devotion to dress. The styles they affect, in their reckless disregard of hygienic rules, strike sturdy German and English matrons with dismay. The latter shiver to behold the gorgeous flimsiness in which such delicate travellers venture to clothe themselves ; and the travellers, in their turn, arch sharp eyebrows and endure twinges of "aromatic pain" whenever these broad-waisted, burly dames cross their vision, in stuffs of coarse woollen and colors too horrible to be borne. At home, our country-woman suffers the more because she is not content to be useless and indolent in all her fine array. Her energy, her intelligence in other matters, must exercise themselves within her house and without it. With strength impaired, she attempts to live the life of the busy worker in a dress that the merest idler would find burdensome and oppressive. The result is a pain and a weariness that lead inevitably to discomfort and disease; but she has not yet learned that, while discomfort is a sin against herself, disease is a sin against God.

The thoughtful, enlightened women of our time have begun to recognize these truths. But they find their pernicious dress imposed upon them as a part of the conventionality into which they are born ; and conventionality is a second nature, which they have been taught to respect far more than Nature at first hand. Indeed, of the latter they as yet know little. Some day, if they persevere in the path which they are now so bravely treading, they will grope their way back to God's original intent in regard to them. Just because their present dress is a part of this tyrannous second nature, do they find it so hard to get rid of it, even when they have declared that they cannot breathe, or walk, or work, or play, or be decently miserable in it. But that knowledge of the laws embodied in her physical being, which woman is acquiring to-day through her study of medicine, and through her forced inquiries into the novel and manifold sufferings she is beginning to experience, together with the new demands of a broader and more active life, lead her to bear with ever-increasing impatience the countless restrictions which her conventional dress imposes upon her. It may be faulty in other respects, it may shock every principle of art, it may demand a wanton expenditure of money and time for its purchase and care; but these appear to her small evils compared with the discomfort and the disease to which it leads.

Thus it has happened that, notwithstanding the many charges which could properly be brought against our prevailing attire, the lectures so far given in this course have concerned themselves almost wholly with its unhealthfulness, — and rightly so. Nothing should overshadow that defect, as nothing can atone for it.

Though it be as perfect in outline and ornament as classic taste can make it, as simple and serviceable as the most energetic worker can desire, a costume has no business to exist, is, indeed, an embodied crime, if it deforms or weakens or tortures the body it pretends to serve. For that should be sacred: it is God's handiwork. He made it as he wished it to be; capable, by wonderful mechanisms, of swift and easy motion; shaped in contours which artists despair of reproducing; and so responsive to our will, so varied in its capacities, so lightly moved from place to place by its own powers, that in its perfect state the soul which inhabits it is almost unconscious of its existence, and knows it only as a source of help and pleasure.

A dress which prevents this human body from ever attaining its natural size and comeliness cannot, however, be simply unhealthful: it must, necessarily, be inartistic, since the highest aspiration of art is to copy and idealize Nature. What opposes Nature can never be really beautiful. And the dress of woman not only hides the form with which she has been endowed, ignoring it as far as possible, and rendering it as if it did not exist, but it shows it still greater disrespect by seeking to interfere with its ordained growth and development. For God's design, it substitutes the design of one of his creatures, — as if the work of the Great Architect could be improved upon! — and strives to shape the body in an artificial mould.

Our costumer does not say, "Here is this outline of trunk and limbs, — let us, in draping it, destroy as little as possible the divine contours into which it grows;" but she says, "Lo, the cages and casings which mine own hands have wrought! Put this body into them, compress it here, add to it there, till it present the likeness of nothing in the heavens above, or in the earth beneath, or in the waters under the earth. Behold it done! This now is my admirable creation, — a woman after my own heart. Do you not admire her?

"What! would you enlarge her casings where they cramp her heart, and curtail her draperies where they clog her feet? Then you despise the loveliness you are too blind to see. You have set up the clownish idol Comfort above Beauty; and Beauty is the divinity we should adore. Go to, unregenerate heathen, who refuse to mingle in our worship! We will have none of you! Depart from our sanctuaries! They who enter here swing censers for ever before the face of our goddess; and with agonies of spirit and great mortification of the flesh do they bow down before our veiled, our corseted, our panniered divinity. Great is her name among the children of men."

And we, the unregenerate heathen, who see

not as they see, must needs retire into caves and dens, and waste places of the earth, and there, in the outer darkness, wail forth this defiant song: "The idol you worship is an impostor, a false god. We scorn to adore her. Lo, on the mountains, free as air, light-footed as the gazelle, roams the true goddess of immortal Beauty! Afar off we behold her as she moves. Her brow is bared to the sweet dews of the morning, and unfading sunshine follows where she treads.'

But the song breaks and quavers, and its feeble echoes threaten to die away upon the hill-tops; while ever upward float full pæans from the crowded idolaters beneath.

Probably no obstacle stand more in the way of a sensible dress-reform, such as health and comfort imperatively demand, than the prevailing notion that any such change must necessarily be hideous, and an offence to the eyes. As if Beauty refused to ally herself with Health and Convenience; and as if they were not the trinity in dress which ought never to be separated!

Indeed, we should pray for a radical change in our attire, if for no other reason than because we believe in beauty. Is not the latter repeatedly outraged in every essential of our present garb?

We hear much from the opponents of such reform concerning the grace of flowing lines; and short skirts they refuse to tolerate, because an important feature of attractive raiment would thus be destroyed. But look at our modern robe. Where be the flowing lines in the flounces, the ruffles, the puffs, the over-skirts, and the bunchings at the waist, which a friend, for lack of a more definite term, has called the great hereafter? Not a single straight sweeping curve from belt to hem; but a terraced, balconied, Chinese pagoda, with gingerbread ornaments confusing its architecture, and meaningless pendants swinging from every support. Can any plain, short skirt be half so bad as that?

If it be true that flowing lines are so excellent a thing, why should they not start from the shoulders, after the manner of the Greek and the Hawaiian dress, and thus secure a longer, more undulating curve for the falling raiment? Or, if that may not be, why not borrow a fashion from the elder Napoleon's court, and extend these lines by terminating the waist just under the arms? Short bodices and long, straight skirts, scant and plain, did not prevent the ladies of the First Empire, Josephine, Hortense, and Madame Récamier, from making themselves fascinating to all beholders; and in that attire Madame de Staël did her deep thinking at Coppet. Health would surely be the gainer by such a change; for whereas now belt and bias tighten around the loose lower ribs and the unprotected stomach, which have no power to resist the outward pressure, then the firm upper ribs would be the parts compressed, and they would stand like a wall of defence around the vital organs within.

But the fashion of to-day will not purchase her vaunted beauties at such a sacrifice. Flowing draperies, admirable as they are, must never be obtained at the expense of the long, tight waist which she takes such infinite pains to mould. That shall survive, if all else perishes. "Lengthen your skirts, by all means," she says, — "the floor is yours, — but never encroach upon the bodice above. I care not if that be the most pernicious feature of the whole attire: it is the one to which I shall most desperately cling."

If girding the body to the closest outline of the form over the region between the ribs and the hips, and there alone, is to remain the one essential accompaniment of a full-dress costume, might we not, at least, have a fixed standard of size for the waist, so that only those who transcend certain bounds may feel compelled to diminish themselves? As it is, no woman, however small, is small enough. Pinching appears to be indispensable. Nature is never allowed to be right as she is.

Not only, then, because those who plead for the retention of woman's present habiliments dodge the great facts of life, and, while prating of the lovely sheen of trailing satins in my lady's drawing-room, forget the physical miseries and inefficiencies of their sex, — of mothers, housekeepers, and workwomen, — must we dissent from their views, but because, in pleading for a fancied beauty such as they see around them, they delay the advent of that higher beauty which must always be consonant with God's laws, and which alone the true artist would recognize.

Those who advocate a real and enduring dress-reform do so not only for the sake of health, but because they cannot forget, through blind adoration of prevailing deformities, in what the true harmonies of form and color consist. One whose life, as an artist, has been given to the study of beauty's laws, arraigns our present dress for "its inconsistency with the just proportions of the human figure; for its prevention of muscular freedom, and consequent falsity to grace and beauty; for its excessive ornamentation, and its introduction of senseless and glaring deformities, which are disgraceful to the wearer, demoralizing to the community, and an outrage to good taste and common sense." This is the dress which it is claimed we cannot change to-day without destroying all the loveliness of female apparel: a dress which so clothes the feet that graceful walking is impossible, and substitutes a hobbling limp in place of that firm and noble carriage which denotes the queen, — *incedit regina;* which prevents the arms from being raised above the head, and keeps them skewered feebly to the side; which obliterates curve of outline and sweep of fold by meaningless and redundant trimming; which exaggerates the bust, humps the hips, pinches the waist, and in every way tends to destroy freedom of motion and symmetry of form.

Where so many enormities exist, one would think that any departure must be for the better. But, despite the contrary notion which prevails, those who are seeking to reconstruct our present dress esteem the beautiful in personal attire — whether in the attire of men or of women — as too important an element to be left to the evolution of chance. The artist whose words I have just quoted, and who is herself a member of that association of ladies in whose behalf I now address you, willingly yields to physiology and hygiene the primal place in the suggestion of remedies for these evils; but she does not forget that "art insists on the recognition of good taste in the construction of dress, not only in excellence of material, in grace of contour, and in harmony of color, but in perfect adaptation to the conditions and necessities of life, claiming that no dress-reform can be speedy, effective, or permanent which ignores the inherent instinct of beauty, no scheme of amendment successful where both beauty and utility do not act in harmonious combination."

It is because we believe in the picturesque, and that no human being has a right to ignore it even in clothes, that we cannot admire the costume which woman adopts to-day. And, were it entirely satisfactory in this respect, we should then feel like remonstrating against that total disregard of beauty which is shown in the dress of the other sex. It is often asserted that they who preach dress-reform for women desire merely that they shall dress like men. Heaven forbid! is our response.

If utility were the only thing to be considered, we might admit that the dress of men is as nearly perfect as it can be made. But it takes no cognizance of those finer needs, of that thirst for beauty for beauty's sake, which God has implanted in our being, and which he has taken such infinite pains to gratify. To this end has he not filled the heavens above us with ever shifting contrasts and harmonies of color, painted the sunrise and the sunset with gold and vermilion, bathed the zenith in softest azure, and spanned the pearly cloud-mists with shaded arches of glowing light?* Has he not decked the earth beneath with a thousand charming hues, given to each flower-petal its own fresh tints and dainty crimpings, mottled every insect's wing with drops of color, and made the plumage of every bird contribute to that feast of beauty which he has spread before our delighted eyes? In such a world of varied and varying loveliness, who shall say that a Quaker garb, or any dull, unchanging uniformity of dress, is in accordance with the divine will? It is a narrow nature that can hold such abnegations to be right and becoming.

The costume which men have chosen for all occasions is an insult to woman's æsthetic tastes. By what privilege, we ask, do they ignore their bounden allegiance to art, and daily afflict our sense of the graces of form and charms of color by the attire they adopt? Have not our eyes rights in this matter as well as theirs? If we have thus far sacrificed every thing to beauty, as we understood it, they have to-day sacrificed every thing to comfort. While we seek to retreat from our one extreme, let them retreat from theirs.

Who that ever sits in the gallery of a crowded ball-room, looking down on the whirling dancers below, is not struck with the ridiculous incongruity in their dress, as they glide in close couples over the floor? The ladies, huge and cylindrical in masses of vaporous tulle, appear smiling and radiant in jewels and garlands and festive array; while the poor little men, black as ebony and straight as clothes-pins, pirouette in bold relief against the spinning cylinders of tulle, clinging to their unsubstantial edges with an anxious look, as if they felt that at any moment a sudden gust might puff them off into the air, or drift them out beyond their bearings. Did we not know the fashions of our modern world, we should suppose that a wedding procession had just broken into a funeral train, and whirled off the mourners to dance a jig. And, judging by their faces, the mourners never forget the bier left halting outside, even when skipping to the sound of the timbrel and lute in the merciless grasp of their captors. But, unlike clothes-pins, the men are not wooden-headed; for, when the music strikes up a quadrille, they show marvellous dexterity in piloting themselves through the vaporous lanes and around their huge partners; and, even in the swift interlacing of the grand-right-and-left, no one of them treads on the lowest, outlying ruffle of the tarlatan mists through which they pick their way. When the music stops with a long scrape from the violin, they are always found bowing in their right places, though they have had to circumnavigate great circles in their devious voyage, to look out for shoals and quicksands on every side, and to tack often in the face of gusty winds and through a chopped sea.

The masculine half of humanity do well to wear about their work a compact, simple, and serviceable dress; but they have no excuse for intruding it upon elegant, social assemblies, and thus robbing them of half their picturesque charm. If men enter such festive scenes, they should don a wedding garment. Nature has not rendered it impossible for them to assume those splendors of the toilet which they are so fond of in us. Once they made themselves magnificent with scarlet velvets slashed with gold, with embroidered ruffs, flashing knee-buckles, and long, powdered hair. Why does not a full-dress occasion demand this of them to-day, as rigorously as it does the trains, the laces, the coiffures of our sex? If it be essential to the brilliancy of the drawing-room that the fall of silken draperies shall reveal their lights and shadows under the blaze of chandeliers, — why, the more of them the better. And if some people must agonize as lay-figures for the sake of others' eyes, let the suffering be equally divided. We will bear our half, let the men bear theirs! Though masculine coat-tails cannot offer us the sweep and shimmer of floating drapery, by trailing on the floor as we trail our robes, their wearers, on state occasions at least, might don the glittering and gorgeous apparel in which they were wont of old to present themselves at the courts of queens, and even in the halls of our provincial assemblies.

Our young friend Antinoüs is a joy to behold, even now, with his classic head rising from a cast-iron shirt collar, and his erect and comely form encased in straight, black pantaloons and a plain frock-coat; but what would he not become in our eyes, could we behold a Tyrolese hat, with a soaring ostrich-feather, shading his brow, and his face smiling a welcome over lace shirt-frills, and a doublet buttoned with diamonds, like that worn by Prince Esterhazy?

But to-day all the picture-making falls to us. We are never supposed to be observers. Men inform us that woman's divine mission is to make herself beautiful; and we, believing all that they tell us, set about adorning ourselves within an inch of our lives, and exist that we may be looked at. Men are handsomer to us than women, — or, at least, Nature meant that they should be: why ought they not, then, to make the most of themselves, in like manner, for our edification? We must go to the opera and the theatre if we would behold man adorned with the perfection of clothes; for there his warbling and strutting are done in the varied and brilliant costumes which other less prosaic times and other less prosaic lands have allowed him to wear.

In every-day life, Claribel's peach-bloom cheeks and lustrous eyes glow and sparkle the more under her veil of gossamer; bright roses wreathe her brow from under her hat; in wavy folds of soft silk she moves before her admirers; and thus, however useless she may otherwise be, she adds a new glory and a diviner beauty to the earth she treads. But unless Antinoüs should become stage-struck, and take to the highway on the boards, in the character of an Italian bandit, or simper as a page in mock drawing-rooms, I shall never see him in the Tyrolese hat and the satin doublet, and he must always appear before me in his second best.

Art obstinately refuses to accommodate herself to man's modern attire. Painters and sculptors keep it out of their pictures and their marbles, and poetry will not recognize it. Were I to write a " Dream of Fair Men," after the manner of Tennyson's " Dream of Fair Women," and take my subjects from the *jeunesse dorée* we see around us, I should find myself put to it to introduce graceful references to their cravats, dress-coats, pantaloons, and tall hats, so as to make them seem either poetic or inspiriting. The only course possible, if I did not wish to rob my heroes of all claims to divinity, would be to ignore their garments altogether. Yet togas, mantles, cloaks, knee-buckles, sandals, cocked hats — these accessories of an elder time — were available in verse. You remember the old poet Herrick's enthusiastic celebrations of his Julia's clothes, — the very same she would wear to-day; and Sir John Suckling says of some one of his court beauties, —

> "Her feet beneath her petticoat
> Like little mice stole in and out,
> As if they feared the light."

So that even petticoats are not alien to song; but could "His boots beneath his pantaloons" in any way get admittance to an immortal poem?

Thus men have had their dress-reform, of a kind we will not emulate. In casting aside their inconvenient fineries, relics of the days when gentlemen were more ornamental than useful, and adopting a suit fitted for business and work, they have forsworn all richness and variety of color and ornament. If women's dress-reform were to mean this, we might well dread the sober look which the world would wear. But beauty must be incorporated into our remodelled garments, so far as it interferes with nothing more important to retain; only let us be sure that it is beauty, and not hideousness. The eternal principles of taste and fitness should be our guides, rather than the changing whims of the mode. Let us also prize the attraction of a strong, well-developed physique as greater than any artificial charm that can be added to it, and devise only that apparelling which is consistent with perfect health. And, while we do this, let us ask that men respect our rights as beauty-loving creatures in the same way that we respect theirs.

It is surely the duty of all human beings to make themselves both useful and beautiful to the extent of their powers; and the obligation to do this rests equally upon the two sexes. But society proceeds on the theory that man has only to be useful, and woman to be beautiful; and that thus their several duties will be well performed. This would be a very comfortable assumption for us, if it were true; but, somehow, a deal of hard drudgery happens to fall to our lot, which no one thinks it his duty to appropriate for the sake of enabling us to fulfil our appointed mission. The work we must do; but we must be as beautiful as possible while doing it. Though forced to play the rôle of the bee, we are never to forget that of the butterfly. So, striving to meet such opposing requirements, we make of our every-day life a continuous, shabby pageant, which brings little pleasure to others or profit to ourselves. We might endeavor to provide the entire æsthetic entertainment demanded by the race, if that were all that were required; but to work and to play at the same time, and in the same troublesome fineries, with never so much as a sorry little farce of the same sort acted for us in return, is to make a dreary failure of the whole.

It is time to have done with such folly. Let us work when we work, and play when we play; and let us seek to do both thoroughly and well. Let us accept the truth that we all have daily tasks,— women as well as men; and let us go to them in the raiment they demand,— raiment strong, warm, cleanly, comfortable; made, too, with all possible regard to beauty, but with that quality kept wholly subordinate and subservient to the capacity for untrammelled action. Then neither the labor nor the laborer will suffer from the dress.

But, work-time over, we may fling utility to the winds, and feed our senses with the sweet satisfactions of beauty and grace. If recreation offers, we will take down our fine feathers from their upper shelves, and, sparing no braveries of color or shape which art suggests and health approves, we will all combine to form a partnership for elegant and elevating enjoyment.

There is no reason why the rich and ornamented garments meet for holiday occasions should not conduce also to comfort and health. But were it otherwise, and could the picturesque element in our apparel be retained only as it was embodied in the cumbrous habiliments of the past, we should say that even then it would be our duty to make some provision for its recognition. Rather than suffer humanity to drape itself continually in dingy hues, with no remembrance of the rich, warm tints, the jewelled radiance, and the soft sheen of light and shadow which once made courtly robes resplendent, and which the old painters — such as Rubens and Titian — loved so well, we should then all agree, with heroic devotion, that for a limited time, and after stated intervals of ease, we would assemble together and make ourselves splendid and miserable for the general good. If each bore his part bravely, and it was fair play, no one would be readier than our dress-reformers to take their chances of surviving with the rest. But they would insist on conditions, and would tolerate no unnecessary risks. There must be short sessions, seasonable hours, spacious, well-warmed, well-ventilated rooms, and no late suppers to tempt them to their death. That none of the effects might be wasted, long mirrors should panel the walls, and a floor smooth and polished repeat the gorgeous scene, as still waters reflect meadow trees in October. Over this glare surface there would be careful hobbling of many guests in high-heeled, sharp-toed slippers; and, when a space was cleared for action, brocaded trains should sweep along before admiring eyes, or whisk about as adroitly as if they belonged to a stage actress who had studied all branches of her profession. Lest any one might become hopelessly involved in their entangling folds, a page should be at hand to reef them when they became unmanageable. Close calculation beforehand would have determined just how much perambulating and attitudinizing ought reasonably to be expected of each contributor; and, having done our duty, we should be free to retire to side stations and survey the other performers. There, in glittering ranks, we should plume the feathers stolen for us from African deserts, shake out wide laces from shivering arms, exalt huge pyramids of powdered locks as if they were horns of the wicked, and stir the deep-hearted, scintillating jewels bound about our brows and the clinking chains upon our wrists. In such trappings, of course we should feel like the veriest puppets, mere inconsequential fragments of the whole combination; but, if it were possible to vivify and inform so much buckram, paste, and dead material, we should do it. Over broad, wired ruffs we would smile radiantly at the velvet coats, the long silk doublets, the drooping frills, and the periwigs of the gallant courtiers before us, and they should smile radiantly in return; and thus the play would be well sustained. Having stipulated that the show should terminate at a fixed hour, we could bear our part without flinching. That hour arriving, a clock-stroke would send us as swiftly to the plain, easy apparel of our daily life, as it sent Cinderella from a royal feast to her kitchen and cold ashes.

Our hungry senses would have had a carnival of color and movement, of courtly grace and beaming compliment, managed according to the most approved co-operative principles, where each one who shared the profits had contributed his proportion of the risks. It would have been in premeditated defiance of the laws of health; but, considering the cause at stake, Hygeia might surely pardon us for our indulgence, provided we paid penance at her shrine for months after in long-sleeved, high-necked flannels, swinging our censers with fur-lined mittens, in strict conformity to calisthenic teaching, and pacing before her altars in sombre walking-suits and the best of Miller's broad-soled boots.

Worshippers of Health though we be, who shall say that we have no regard for Beauty, when, if all friends forsook her, we would lay such homage at her feet? But she will never exact of us this last measure of devotion. She prefers to leave behind her the stilted magnificence of the past, and to mingle with us in our daily toil and daily pleasures. Her touch shall hereafter brighten the coarse robe of the workwoman, as well as the mantle of the queen; and, when she summons us to her dainty banquets, we shall find Simplicity and Health among her guests.

While we bewail the imperfections of clothes, as now worn by men and women, we do not sorrow as those without hope. Already indications appear that man's attire has reached its acme of ugliness, and that the reaction towards adornment and color has begun. If the feather he sticks in his new hat-band is a very tiny one, and worn with a half-shamed air, it is still there, a veritable bit of color and grace, and useful for nothing else. It is but a line of piping, but it carries a streak of scarlet through the gray uniformity of his winter riding-coat; and the gay posy pinned into his button-hole is another step towards the happy mean which lies between mere comfort on the one hand and mere beauty on the other.

And, looking at the general tendency of the late fashions devised for women, the prospect seems equally encouraging for them. If a wanton luxuriance of trimming runs riot over hampering train and torturing bodice, there is likewise provision for higher and purer tastes, and the severe finds a place beside the ornate. Simplicity of adornment, unbroken lines, looseness at the waist if you will, — what more can you hope for to-day? Mantua-makers tell us that the late Parisian fashion-plates retain straight redingotes for women, and even herald the return of short skirts; and that all these may be plain to a degree. Beneath such an exterior, what hinders you from being as comfortable as you can ever be under the old *régime* of skirts and bodices? Ungird your waistbands, and put on your suspenders: who shall be the wiser?

Nor would we forget the substantial gains of the past ten years. Waterproof cloaks and rubber boots have been vouchsafed us, in recognition of the fact that women have acquired regular occupations outside their homes, and must go abroad in rainy weather as well as in fair. Corsets, bad as they are, are no longer laced with the aid of the bedpost, nor worn at night. Low necks and short sleeves are seldom displayed at balls and parties; and let us believe that, for the sake of common decency, they will rarely be seen there again. A few years ago we should have cited close coat-sleeves, comfortable boots, short walking-dresses, and hats in lieu of bonnets, as further proofs that the world of fashion was swinging steadily towards the millennium. But, alas! since then we have seemed to be returning towards chaos and old night; for flowing sleeves, high-heeled boots, and trailing skirts for the street have come in again, and, however brief their reign, they have shown us that women are as ready as ever to freeze their arms, to torture and deform their feet, and to sit enveloped in breadths of drapery which have swept the public sidewalks for a mile. The worse for the credit of women and the credit of fashion! It teaches us to put no faith in any fair promises that the fickle goddess may make. If to-day she offers us plain and sensible habiliments, to-morrow she will lead us a terrible life again, with her flutings and flouncings. She is not converted to the side of dress-reform, only trying her hand at oddities. And, if we should call in her aid to help along our thoughtful work, she would jilt us just as it was well under way. Could we create the dress of which we dream, and, securing Mme. Demorest and the fashion magazines, astonish the world with a *coup d'état* which should make women appear for once clad like reasonable beings, by what force could we compel them to retain this mode longer than the season which produced it? Laws, to endure in a republic, must be approved by the people who submit to them. If the majority of its wearers see no other reason for the adoption of a costume than that they find it in their fashion-books, it will be abandoned when another supersedes it there.

Here is the obstacle which is to be overcome, if we would look for any effectual and enduring dress-reform among the women of to-day, such as the good of our American society now demands. It cannot be imposed upon any one: its wearers must desire it for themselves. They must desire it, moreover, for reasons which shall render it necessary to retain it as a permanency.

These reasons will be, first, a respect for their physical natures, and an enlightened belief that their own bodily weakness and inefficiency are chiefly due to the injurious effects of wearing the present dress. The second reason will be an artistic perception of what true beauty is, and a desire to conform to it, independently of any arbitrary rules of taste. In short, they must learn

Nature's laws, and respect them. The few who have done so hitherto have been powerless to arouse the many. Who shall become to her sisters the valiant and persuasive apostle of the divinity of the body? Who shall reveal to them the eternal harmonies of form and color, so that they shall listen, and be ready to obey?

That desirable improvement in the dress both of women and men which art enjoins will surely come in time, if we can wait patiently for it. Such a general knowledge of beauty's laws, and such a deference to their behests as it implies, must be a slow growth; for it is nothing short of the enlightenment of the whole people as to what constitutes grace of form, harmony of color, and adaptability to conditions of life. The importance of this art-education, too long ignored and despised in our Puritan New World communities, has been at length recognized by our public authorities in such a manner that it cannot fail to be well provided for hereafter. With drawing taught in every one of our public schools, with the establishment of schools of design for mechanics in our principal cities, and free lectures delivered upon the elements of beauty, and with the opening of museums of painting and statuary to cultivate the taste of all observers, we must find hereafter not only a perceptible improvement in our manufactured articles of household use, but also in the outlines and the details of our daily dress.

And we see further hope in the fact that as the making of our garments tends to pass more and more into the hands of professional workwomen, so the designing of them will, in consequence, fall to persons trained for such tasks. Woman's time is fast becoming valuable to her for other labors than the devising at home of all the articles that she wears ; and she now seeks to find them ready-made for her use, as man finds his apparel. The supply of finished dresses, and underclothing of all descriptions, in our stores, is a feature of the past five years, and is destined to work a revolution not only in woman's work but in woman's appearance. It may, perhaps, tend to greater sameness of attire, but it must tend also to better taste, since individual ignorance will not be forced to embody and illustrate itself in every article which it wears. But no influence can ever destroy the peculiar character which each one confers upon her attire, or prevent a revelation of that delicate and cultured taste which shows itself in the tie of a neck-ribbon and the arrangement of the simplest details.

When, by such means, true beauty becomes familiar, it will be understood; and then it will work itself out into such a readjustment of the essential outlines of our dress as may adapt them to the untrammelled growth and motion of the human figure, whose native grace it will have learned to revere. Thus, slowly but surely, will Art take to herself the right to shape and adorn the material with which we are clothed.

We have reason to believe that instruction as to what constitutes a healthful and serviceable costume will be more speedy, and its beneficial results more immediate. A sad experience of physical ailments will lead women more and more to an inquiry concerning the causes of disease; physicians of their own sex will be able and ready to enlighten them as to the tendency of fashions which are now heedlessly adopted; and the liberal education which they will hereafter receive at school must result in an intelligent comprehension of Nature's laws. They will then desire such a reform as has been advocated, not because it has become, or can become, suddenly fashionable, but because they shrink from subjecting themselves again to ligatures and burdens which can only weaken and oppress.

In this work we ought to have men for allies instead of opponents; for they have themselves struggled out of the same wilderness where we are now wandering. And could they be made to realize the daily and hourly discomfort inflicted by the clothes they admire so much, could they know what hindrances these are to us, and what time and thought we spend upon them, they would cease to ridicule any attempt at dress-reform, and would rather strive to lend it all possible aid and encouragement. But many of them appear amazed that any thing has been found wrong with the drapery in which lovely woman is enshrined; while others, firmly believing that in order to make woman healthy in body it is absolutely necessary to make her hideous in apparel, hold it advisable for their sisters to continue to commit slow suicide in the service of Art. Though they positively declined to do this themselves, when they fashioned their present attire, they are yet ready, like Artemas Ward, to sacrifice all their female relatives in that cause.

Were I an emperor, absolute as any Shah, it would be my sovereign pleasure to decree that the men of my kingdom should wear women's clothes for a day, and that the women should wear those of the men. For one day only. It would not be long before something would be done; for the close of that memorable time would behold a race of groaning athletes, giving thanks for their escape from the strange bondage and drawing great breaths of deliverance, while the wailing of the women at their return to the old fetters would be heart-rending to hear. Then the nation would pause from its consideration of lesser evils, and would set at work in good earnest to eradicate this.

But since we can hope for no such aid and comfort, upon what shall we rely? While the sure growth of general intelligence, of which I have spoken, must tend to better fashions, the demands of business, now that women have gone from the home to the workshop and the counter, will force them in time so to attire themselves as not to impair the market value of their labors.

And only such agencies will prove effective in producing greater economy in dress. When woman learns the value of money by laboring directly for it, or when she is informed beforehand of the precise amount of her yearly supplies and feels bound to apportion them according to her needs, when she has opportunities offered her for a nobler competition with her associates than that to which she is now restricted, and which consists in mere personal display, and when, by understanding and respecting Nature, she is led to assign to conventionalism a secondary place, she will then, doubtless, limit her expenditures to her means, and will employ her powers in more profitable toil than in fashioning an endless variety of hideous and cruel garments wherewith to bedeck and torture her suffering frame.

Although the varied influences now at work in the society around us must inevitably result, sooner or later, in a sensible reconstruction of dress, we should do our utmost to make the transition as speedy as possible, in order that our sisters may be spared all needless suffering and inefficiency. Much can be done by the direct appeals of those who are zealous in this cause to those who are not, by the mighty force of example, in rendering pernicious fashions unpopular, and in holding to those which are good; and, especially, by the instruction of the young women of our schools in the inflexible laws of their being, concerning which they are now so lamentably ignorant, and a knowledge of which is so essential to the physical well-being of themselves, their families, and remote posterity.

Of all the seed that can be scattered by the wayside, none will bear such promise of fruit as that which shall fall upon young minds. It is with the girls that this reformation must begin, if it is to prove effectual. We older women, and all like us, however strong and well we may think ourselves, are, at the best, little better than physical wrecks, capable of repairs more or less thorough, but still hopelessly damaged by the ignorance of ourselves and of our time. What we might have been in our physiques, had we been properly trained and clothed from childhood, we can never know. But the girls of to-day should be saved before they have learned to wear the woman's dress, with its countless abominations, that they may be enabled to grow up untrammelled, vigorous, and happy, to show the world a nobler womanhood and a nobler race of children than our country offers now. Practical teaching of this sort the pupils of our schools seem glad to hear and enthusiastic to follow. In large cities its need is imperative.

And just now it is especially important, not only to the physical but to the mental well-being of our girls and women, that some thorough dress-reform should be effected. It is the bodily weakness, resulting so largely from their attire, which has become the chief argument for dwarfing and restraining their intellectual growth.

Admitting, as we must, that the undoubted ill-health of our countrywomen is a national injury and a national disgrace, we should feel called upon as patriotic citizens and as philanthropists to do every thing in our power to remove the causes which induce it. No one habit of American life can be held responsible for it; the agencies are manifold which convert so many of our vigorous girls into suffering invalids before they have fairly grown into women: but, if there be one agency worthy to be emphasized above all others, I believe it to be our present pernicious style of dress. A physician who could attribute the sad decay of our young women to excessive and continuous study, must be ignorant of very much of what constitutes the daily life of those of whom he speaks ; and I protest against that explanation of the prevailing invalidism which has lately been given, and which is so eagerly caught at and proclaimed by those who are at heart opposed to every belief which tends to develop woman into something more than a merely physical being, valuable to society not for her own sake, but only because she is the mother of an order of beings superior to herself. The fact that girls, upon whose muscular and nervous systems such a peculiar strain is to come in their after-lives, are suffered to do nothing in youth which shall strengthen those muscles and tone those nerves ; that half-grown limbs, unfilled lungs, sluggish livers, pinched stomachs, and distorted wombs are carefully cultivated by the corsets and tight waists in which we encase their developing bodies ; and that sedentary habits, bad air, and poor appetites are given them as a daily portion when we keep them in-doors and seek to train them into presentable young ladies, — argues nothing against the native endurance of their physical frames, but rather tends to show that there must be an extraordinary amount of vitality and recuperative power in what refuses so obstinately to be destroyed. It is a ludicrous mistake to suppose that a few sporadic cases of injudicious study in the few female colleges of the land can be held accountable for the general ill-health of our women. Had any masculine physician who entertains that idea ever made a study of the full feminine regalia in which his delicate patients sit enveloped when they come to consult his professional skill, he would have found, in chilled and encumbered limbs, dragging skirts, overheated abdomen, compressed waist, and hot and burdened head, a better explanation of that state of things which he and all well-wishers of our country and our race must lament. It is not that boys and girls are trained too much alike mentally, but that they are trained too much unlike physically, which works the harm. Not too much knowledge of astronomy and mathematics, but too little knowledge of the laws of life, is what proves fatal to our young women. The remedy for their weakness is to be sought, not by enfeebling the mind till mind and body correspond, but by strengthening the body, through intelligent obedience to its laws, so that mind and body can both attain their perfect stature.

When the instruction so much needed on vital matters is furnished to our girls by their parents and teachers, they will abandon for ever the style of apparel which now works such disastrous results; and then, with proper clothing and proper training, they will be enabled to grow up, not into those strange, unfeminized beings, ashamed of their sex, of whom some writers morbidly dream, but into strong-bodied, strong-limbed, clear-headed, warm-hearted, rosy, happy women, proud of their womanhood, surrounded by husband and children, if they prefer a domestic life, but held in equal honor and esteem, if, for any reasons which may seem to them good, they choose to devote themselves, with self-reliant energies, to other labors for their race.

If any lady has become convinced of a radical and pernicious error in the construction of her dress, and desires to reform it altogether, let her not wait till a costume which is both healthful and elegant shall spring into being, to serve as a model. Individual thought and effort must be expended, if individual wants are to be met. No regulation-suit can be offered which would prove acceptable to all. What one finds agreeable in material and make, another is sure she could not tolerate. Therefore each one will need to work out her own physical salvation with patience and devotion. But the result will justify her pains.

In the first place, she must divest herself of the common notion that a dress-reform necessarily and primarily means a marked change in the outer garment, — the "dress," technically so called, — and in that alone. The under-garments are the chief offenders; and it is far more important that they should be remodelled than that any change should be made in the external covering.

Indeed, there is no necessity for any dress-reformer to play the rôle of a martyr by appearing in a singular and conspicuous garb, unless she chooses to do so. Bring me your latest fashionable costumes, — the dresses just fresh from Paris, made by Worth himself, if you will, — and I will pick one from among them beneath which it shall be possible to dress a woman in almost perfect conformity to the laws of health. Not one binding shall be needed at the waist.

And if any have succeeded in reconstructing their clothing so as to render it in harmony with hygienic and æsthetic laws, they should endeavor to benefit others by offering practical suggestions, and by extending the advantages they have derived from their own troublous experiences and final triumphs. For dress-reformers must never become so thoroughly comfortable that they will not remember those who are still in the bonds of corsets and waistbands, as bound with them.

Such work, for ourselves and for others, will hasten the day when woman shall be more than her dress ; when the latter, from being a master shall become a servant, and man's work be held less admirable than that of God.

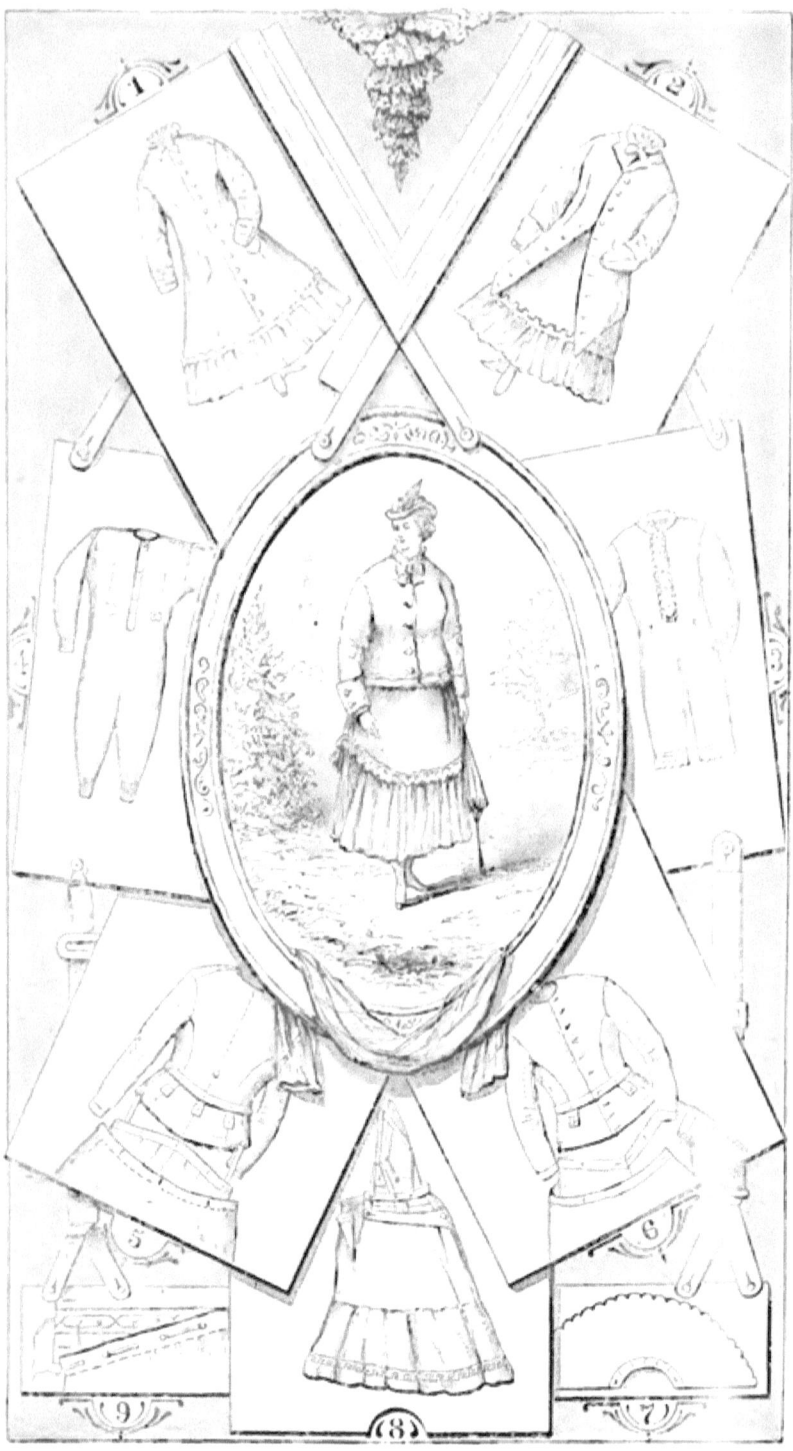

APPENDIX.

APPENDIX.

The common and serious charge brought against all reformers is that they are always ready to pull the world to pieces, and very slow to reconstruct it again. And yet a dissatisfaction with existing evils must precede the desire for any thing better, and is the one step without which subsequent advance would be impossible. To create a "divine discontent" with reigning abuses is to prepare the way for their ultimate overthrow.

But, in the matter before us, immediate remedies are so desirable and important that those who are calling attention to pernicious features of the present apparel feel impelled to provide some acceptable substitute. It is their wish to show not only why, but how, a dress-reform should be made.

Accordingly, the preceding lectures have not merely demonstrated that all the devices of the female mind as to personal attire have been evil, and that continually, but they have sought to indicate what other and better garments should now be adopted. Further detailed and definite suggestions concerning the changes that need to be made will be found in this Appendix, which is intended to supplement the words of the physicians, and which will contain such directions for the proper fashioning and adjustment of the under dress, and for the improvement of the whole apparel, as may render its pages of practical value.

"This book is for the good, and not for the bad," wrote the "child" Bettine, in her crude English, at the beginning of that volume of Correspondence which she was struggling so hard to translate from her native German into a foreign tongue. And so I may say at starting that this Appendix is for earnest and sensible women who are seeking to reconstruct their clothing upon true principles of physiology and art: it is not for triflers, who have no interest in reform beyond the diverting literature it supplies. Doubtless many such will peruse it; but, if they are warned at the entrance that it is dangerous passing here, their delicate sensibilities cannot bring a complaint for any injuries they may receive. A description of novel garments, to be of any service, must be minute and explicit; and, since I am writing for women, the designations in common use among them will be employed, without foolish circumlocutions.

The unreasoning prejudices of the general public are so strong against any radical change in the present appearance of woman's dress, that they could not fail to conquer, at last, whatever bravery and intelligence might to-day be displayed in the adoption of a wholly new and singular garb. It would, therefore, seem wise to conciliate, as far as possible, these powerful prejudices; while, at the same time, effecting that thorough reform in the structure of the underwear, and those modifications of the outer dress, which health imperatively demands. So long as the entire underwear remains ill-formed and ill-adjusted, no fitness in the externals can confer the ease and freedom which our clothing should secure. If we would gain essential improvements that are vital to good health and long life, we must decide to attempt no specious and superficial reform, nor one, however thorough, that would inevitably come to a speedy and disastrous end. Great care and much deliberation are needed in devising a style of dress that shall be loose, light, and of uniform thickness, while it retains the general and obvious features of the costume of our time.

But the problem is one which patient and continued efforts have at length solved. Many ladies, interested in the work, have devoted their ingenuity and practised skill to the invention of a simple, healthful, and complete suit of underwear, which may take the place of our present objectionable styles, and they have succeeded in obtaining it. The forms and combinations of the ordinary garments have been well considered, and their evils and advantages clearly defined. As the result of this examination, we have been led to abandon altogether some of the garments commonly worn, as hopelessly bad, to modify others, to recommend a few hitherto but little known, and to invent some that are wholly new and strange. These last have been evolved by slow stages from what were at first but floating visions of hygienic principles embodied in clothes; and these visions have thus assumed a local habitation, and even a name, among the regenerated garments of the new dispensation. Whoever has given herself to the cutting, basting, fitting, and altering, which are needed for the final realization of such dreams, will allow the inventors to survey their triumphs with pardonable pride. It is no idle thing to wrestle with cotton cloth and come off the victor.

These selections and successes have been of sufficient number to present a variety of forms for the choice of would-be dress-reformers; for even they have prejudices to be humored and individual tastes to be met. No two of them were ever known to choose the same outfit, in all its combinations and details; though all must agree on the general principles to which every article should conform.

Before proceeding to particularize, let me define these few hygienic principles, and state, also, the precise objects which have been held in view in our attempted reconstruction of dress.

First, and most important, the vital organs situated in central regions of the body must be allowed unimpeded action.

Second, a uniform temperature of the body must be preserved.

Third, weight must be reduced to a minimum.

Fourth, the shoulders, and not the hips, must serve as the base of support.

The first will require that all tight-fitting waists of whatever sort, whether in under or outer wear, and all tight ligatures about the waist, be entirely removed.

The second will require that the clothing be made of the same thickness throughout, in order that the uniform temperature natural to the body may not be disturbed and destroyed.

APPENDIX.

There must be no less on the limbs than on the trunk; no less on the shoulders than on the waist; and no more below the waist than above. I have said that there should be no less on the limbs; but there should really be more, since, being of great length in proportion to their diameter, and disconnected with the main part of the body save at one end, they offer a large extent of surface for the radiation of heat, and therefore tend to become colder than other sections. They are remote from the vital organs whose constant action increases the temperature of surrounding parts; and the blood, on which the system chiefly depends for its warmth, has to traverse long distances in order to reach their extremities, and must suffer a gradual diminution of heat as it flows outward. This is especially true of the feet. They are very far from the centre, and move upon the ground, in the lowest and coldest stratum of the atmosphere. Thus the blood in them is liable to chills, and these are transmitted to portions above. Special pains must therefore be taken to protect the feet with warm coverings, to elevate their soles above the ground, by many layers of stout leather rendered nearly impervious to cold and moisture, and, also, to give as much freedom to the movements of the feet beneath their coverings as ease in walking will allow. By so doing, we shall permit the vital currents within the feet to flow freely back and forth from the heart. So much for the limbs. On the trunk of the body, all the upper garments should extend from the neck only so far as to meet the lower garments; otherwise, we shall have the neck and shoulders cold, and the pelvic region overheated. Every thickness of cloth which covers the trunk should furnish sleeves and drawers for the limbs; and additional coverings should be had for the legs and feet, to be worn in the outer air.

The third principle will require that the skirts, which do now, and must ever, so long as they are worn, contribute the chief weight of our clothing, shall be made as few, as short, as scant, as sparingly trimmed, as good looks will permit.

The fourth will require that all the lower garments be attached to the upper garments, or that they have separate and special supports of their own passing over the shoulders.

If we try our present attire by these requirements, we shall see clearly why it fails to embody, or even to recognize, the elementary principles that have been stated, and why radical changes must be made.

Our ordinary dress provides two tight-fitting waists, either of which suffices to force the vital organs beneath it out of place and upon each other. In the underwear, the corset reigns supreme; in the outer dress, the plain or biased waist is usually buttoned as tightly over the corset as it can possibly be drawn. Beneath such compressions, what becomes of the action of the diaphragm, the lungs, the heart, and the stomach? Then, again, every one of the lower garments has a binding fastened around the waist, and this binding is composed of a straight piece of cloth folded double. Drawers, underskirts, balmoral, dress skirt, over-skirt, dress-waist, and belt, furnish, accordingly, sixteen layers of cloth girding the stomach and the yielding muscles situated in that region. These bands are all placed one directly over the other on the same line, and are usually made as tight as they can be buttoned; so that a belt of iron, two inches wide, welded close about the body, could hardly be more unyielding. In such attire, if any one escapes weak lungs, short breath, palpitation of the heart, liver-complaint, and indigestion, it is by a special interposition of the higher powers in her individual case. Who shall say this is not an age of miracles? Thus the first hygienic rule is set at naught.

The second rule, which enjoins uniform temperature, meets with like respect. The limbs have not half the amount of covering which is put upon the trunk of the body. Many garments have no sleeves; and what sleeves there are either come to an end a few inches below the shoulder, or they are loose and flowing at the wrists, so as to expose the arm as far as the elbow to the cold air. As to the legs, the clothing, which should increase in direct ratio to the distance from the body to the feet, diminishes in the same ratio. Thin drawers, thinner stockings, and wind-blown skirts which keep up constant currents of air, supply little warmth to the limbs beneath. The feet, half-clad, and pinched in tight boots, are chilled in consequence. The trunk of the body has as many varied zones of temperature as the planet it inhabits. Its frigid zone is above, on the shoulders and the chest; for, although the dress-waist extends from the neck to the waist, most, if not all, of the garments worn beneath it are low-necked. The temperate zone lies between the shoulders and the belt; for that region receives the additional coverings of under-vest, corset, and chemise. The torrid zone begins with the belts and bands, and extends to the limbs below; for all the upper garments are continued below the belt, and all the lower garments, the drawers and skirts, come up as far as the belt: so that the clothing over the whole pelvic region must be at least double what it is over any other section. But it is more than double, it is quadruple; for the tops of all these lower garments have a superfluous fulness of material which is brought into the binding by gathers or by plaits. These are especially abundant at the back, over the spine, where one of the centres of the nervous system is situated, and where the kidneys lie. When to this excess of cloth is added a panier and sash-bows, we can understand why deadly torrid heats prevail in that region, and why the worst consequences follow. The result is stated by a physician to be "a chronic inflammation of the internal organs, — mother of a hundred ills that afflict women."

The weight of our clothing increases every year; and, if much more is added, women will be compelled to maintain a sitting posture the greater part of the time, in order to render their dress endurable. *Sedet, æternumque sedebit, infelix Theseus.* Skirts, in their best estate, require considerable cloth; and the greater number of them are made of the heaviest material commonly worn, — viz., cotton cloth, with the addition of trimmings. The dress skirt is long, and doubled by an over-skirt; and, in place of the simple gimps and braids and the few ruffles once used for adorning them, the material of the dress is heaped upon the breadths, in the form of puffs, flounces, and plaits. Add to this burden heavy cotton linings, facings, and "skirt-protectors" at the bottom, and the weight can only be described as enormous.

Then, as to the suspension of clothing from the shoulders. Of course, all the garments worn above the waist hang from the shoulders by necessity; but all the lower garments, as now worn, hang from the hips, and have no connection whatever with any piece above. Many would fain believe that the hips are the proper points of support; but the testimony of all medical intelligence on this subject is clear and indisputable. Our four physicians were unanimous and emphatic in their declarations that the hips should be relieved of all weight; and no physician has been found anywhere to advocate a different view. One says in a published paper, "No description can give any adequate idea of the evils consequent upon wearing skirts hanging from the hips;" and still another says, "Women carry their clothing suspended mainly from their hips; and, as the clothes press by their weight upon the soft abdominal walls, they cause displacement of the internal organs." It is this dragging down — not upon the hip-bones themselves, but upon the front and unprotected portions of the body which they enclose — that produces the chief harm. Even the dress skirts now force the hips to carry their excessive burdens. Formerly, as we all remember, each dress had but one skirt, and this was invariably sewed to the waist. Thus it hung directly from the shoulders, provided the bodice was loose enough to allow any tension to extend to the regions above. When the dress skirts were first made as separate garments, and put into bindings of their own, the arrangement was thought to add greatly to convenience, but it has proved one of the most pernicious features of our present style of dress.

The facts already stated must convince my

readers that the attire now worn by women, in its utter disregard of physiological laws, is not only an injury to themselves, but an insult to their Maker, and an undoubted abomination in his sight.

Some garments are found to be wholly irreconcilable with these laws, and should therefore be dispensed with altogether. Of these, the most important are the corset and the chemise. Since they are the very two without which the average female mind will find it impossible to conceive of further existence upon this terrestrial sphere, I shall do well to pause, and state clearly wherein their objectionable characteristics lie, and why they are past remedy.

Corset. — Concerning the evils of this garment, it would seem that enough has already been said. Physicians have always denounced it as most pernicious, and have refused to compromise with it in any of its forms. But, in spite of these protests, women still cling to it, and still declare that they must wear it or perish. It holds its place because of one or two plausible arguments in its favor, which are not met and reasoned away, but suffered to remain unrecognized and unrefuted. Since they prove so powerful, they ought to receive more serious attention.

Enfeebled by past errors in dress, and with muscles rendered incapable, by enforced inaction, of doing their appointed work, wearers of the corset assert that it is absolutely essential to the support of the body, and that without it they would collapse into an uncertain shape, with neither contours nor comeliness. They claim that its upper portion is needed for the support of the bust, and that its lower portion serves as a shield and protector for the abdomen, so that heavy skirts do not drag them to the earth.

In short, had no human being been bright enough for the invention of this garment, one-half of God's humanity must have been a hopeless failure. He was able, it appears, to construct man so that he should be equal to the requirements of the life conferred upon him; but woman came forth from his hand wholly incompetent to maintain herself erect, or to discharge the daily duties enjoined upon her. Fortunately, some one of his creatures, seeing the deficiency, succeeded in supplementing his work. Thus one skeleton sufficed for men; but for women it had to be propped up externally by another skeleton strapped about it. Or, in other words, Nature made man, but Nature plus Art made woman: take away Art, and she becomes chaos, — "a shapeless form and void." Does any one believe that, when the Creator gave to women their forms, he did not also give them the muscles which its proper maintenance would require?

Tie a strong, healthy arm to a board, and keep it there for months; then remove its artificial prop. The arm cannot lift itself; it falls helpless at the side: *ergo*, never take the arm from the board, and it will never be weak. If an undue fulness of bust needs support, let the support come from above, and not from below. Portly Roman matrons girded up their breasts from shoulder to shoulder, and never dreamed of a corset.* For them, support did not imply, or necessitate, compression of the waist. Cannot modern women equal them in ingenuity and good sense? Cases which would require such provision are rarer than they seem. The great majority of women, growing up without corsets, would find them wholly useless. In strength the body would prove sufficient unto itself. To doubt this is to doubt divine foresight, power, or benevolence.

It is true that corsets prevent one from feeling, at every motion, the pull and drag of each separate binding at the waist; but it is as Nature

---

* "Stays for compressing the form into an unnatural appearance of slimness were not known to the ancients, and would have been an abomination in their eyes. In one of the plays of Terence, a severe censure is conveyed on so unnatural a taste, which is confirmed by all the monuments of art. Still we should be in error if we supposed a girl in those days, even though *vincto pectore*, was provided with stays. All they had was a bosom-band (*strophium mammillare*), for the purpose of elevating the bosom, and also perhaps to confine in some degree the *nimius tumor*. We must not confound with this the *fascia pectoralis*, which was merely worn to confine the breast in its growth, and was, consequently, not a part of the usual dress. The *strophium* was placed over the inner *tunica*, and was usually made of leather."—*Anthon's Roman Antiquities*.

relieves us from the sensation of pain when it becomes excruciating. Numbness deadens the nerves; and corsets deaden sensation by a compression which induces partial numbness. The whole body beneath them being crowded together till its parts are incapable of much distinct motion among themselves, no one portion is conscious of more discomfort than the rest. This is why they render the skirt-bands endurable. Give up the corset, and retain all other garments as previously worn, and the clothing becomes insupportable. The remedy is not to replace the compress as before, but to modify the remainder of the clothing till it is brought into some accordance with physiological laws. To reduce the weight of the skirts, to enlarge their bindings and suspend them from above, would be the only sensible cure. The corset would then be a superfluity, if it were nothing worse.

But many say, the corset is only bad when it is worn tight; loosen it, and it can do no harm; its abuse, and not its use should be condemned.

This statement is inadmissible. A corset is always bad, whether laced or not. Its very structure necessitates a pinching of the waist in front, even when no strings are tied : for, by many slender gores artfully woven into the cloth, it is given the shape of an hour-glass ; and, if it is tight enough to retain its place at all, it must enforce this shape upon the yielding body beneath, with the stomach crowded into the neck of the glass.

It is not thus that Nature models her human beings, whether women or men. The trunk of the body resembles an Egyptian column, with the greatest girth about the middle. The lower ribs spread out, and enclose a larger space than the upper ribs, as a glance at page 47 will show. Below these floating ribs, there are no bones whatever at the waist, if we except the spine behind, which serves as a connecting line between the upper and lower portions of the framework. The reason for this is apparent. No bones can be trusted over this region, lest they impede the full and free action of vital organs beneath. Soft flesh and elastic muscles are the only wrapping allowed. Thus Nature has left the body. Should not this teach woman how to construct the covering she adds to this part of her system? But what does she do? Taking advantage of its yielding character, she crowds this section inward, instead of permitting it to expand outward; and girds and laces and binds and tortures it, till it is smaller than any bones would compel it to be. What should be the base of the pyramid is converted into its apex. While it was designed that all human beings should be larger below the ribs than below the arms, women have so re-formed themselves that they would be ashamed to resemble the Venus of Milo, or even the petite and mincing Venus de Medici. They go, however, in their best "glove-fitting" French corsets, to study those famous marbles in galleries of art, and express unbounded admiration for the superb loveliness of their forms, and the wonderful fidelity to nature which ancient sculptors displayed.

Furthermore, the trunk of the body is meant

to be flexible, to bend backward and forward easily within certain limits. To allow this, the one bone which runs its entire length — the backbone — is broken wholly apart at every inch of its extent, and a supple joint inserted. But the corset, by means of two long, stiff whalebones behind, and two long metal bars in front, forces the body to remain as inflexible throughout that section as if, for half a yard, it were strapped firmly between two iron bars. The lower cells of the lungs would expand, the bars say, No; the stomach would rise and fall as the heart throbs, the bars say, No; the body would bend backward and forward at the waist in a hundred slight movements, the bars say, No: keep to your line; thus far shalt thou go, and no farther. But Nature is both sly and strong, and she loves her way. She will outwit artifice in the long run, whatever it may cost her. The iron bars defy her power; but, by days and months of steady pressure, thrusting them back from her persistently, she forces them to bend. This done, the human hand, that could not curve them at first, cannot make them straight again. Nature has moulded her barriers to accommodate, in some measure, her own needs; and, when they are replaced with new, she sets herself again to the work.

But it is said, "You can improve corsets in several ways, and render them harmless." Without doubt there is a choice in their varieties. Many women, I am aware, rise up and call Madame Foye blessed; and there are manufacturers who proclaim "comfort corsets," with shoulder-straps above, and buttons for stocking-suspenders below, and lacings under the arm as well as behind, and other contrivances intended to render them worthy to be worn in the millennium. None, however, banish the iron in front, which is one of their worst features. But these efforts to improve corsets reveal a determination on the part of their makers to keep them in vogue. All they can do, however, will furnish but trifling mitigations of an evil which can never be converted into a good. A witty writer once discoursed on the "total depravity of material things;" and, if one thing can be more totally depraved than another, that thing is the corset. By and by, as intelligence increases, and the practices of ignorance disappear, the compression of the waist now practised by European and American women will be held to be as ridiculous and far more pernicious than the compression of the feet practised by the Chinese. Indeed, our heathen sisters must appear far more sensible than we; for their favorite torture affects only a remote and comparatively unimportant part of the body, while ours is a torture of the trunk at its very centre, where the springs of life are certain to be weakened and diseased.

One of the strongest reasons for the general adoption of the corset — though it is one not commonly avowed — is the belief that it conduces to beauty and symmetry of figure. Slender forms are usually praised, and chiefly because they are associated with the litheness and the undeveloped graces of youth. But a pinched waist cannot make a slender form, or give the appearance of one, if above and below there be breadth and thickness which no efforts can diminish. Indeed, broad shoulders and a full chest only appear the larger by contrast with the slight span of a girded waist; and thus they become more conspicuous from the attempt made to conceal them. The waist itself, lacking the easy, varied motion and the peculiar shape which Nature gives, deceives no one as to the cause of its small dimensions; and the poor sufferer, who would fain pass for a wand-like sylph, tortures herself in vain, and has only her pains for her labor. Although all men disclaim any liking for an unnaturally small waist, all women persist in believing that a wasp-like appearance, at whatever age, and under whatever conditions, is sure to render them lovelier in the eyes of their admirers. Mature matrons should have a look of stability, and that dignity of presence and carriage which only a portly, well-developed person seems to confer. Such a mien is as much the beauty of middle age, as slenderness is the beauty of youth. And a large, robust woman never looks so well-shaped and comely as when waist and shoulders retain the proportionate size which Nature gave.

But the defenders of the garment in question are found ready to dispute every inch of ground on their forced retreat. They say, " The corsets now worn are surely a great improvement on those of the past: how much more delicate and flexible they are than the stanch buckram stays of a hundred years ago!" Before me lies a pair of such stays, looking as bright and new as if made yesterday, and yet known to have been worn in the year 1787, by a country squire's wife, in what was then the province of Maine. They are home-made, stout, and formidable. Between an external covering of firm green worsted cloth, of unknown make, and a lining of white linen, bound together on the edges with white kid, are ranged stiff whalebones, — over a hundred in number, by actual count, — placed close beside each other, with rows of white stitching set faithfully between. Seven segments, or gores, divide the stays from top to bottom, and give them that clumsy shape for which, no doubt, they were chiefly prized. In Hogarth's pictures we see their exact prototypes. Glancing at them, one would say that they were incomparably worse than the corset of to-day. They are stiff and thick and heavy, laced behind with a leather string, still tied to the eyelet-holes, while a broad wooden busk keeps the long front as straight and imposing as appear the bodices of Copley's painted ladies, or that of Queen Elizabeth herself. In our modern corset, it is not all stiffening: there are lucid intervals between the bones, where cotton cloth pure and simple has a place; but these are in reality a whalebone cuirass, with a hundred vertical joints. Yet, terrible as they look, there is no ground for supposing that they proved fatal to their wearer. Her great-grand-daughter, who writes this, knows little concerning her, save that she lived honored and respected in spite of her stays; and if she died in consequence of them, it was at a goodly age, and the cause of her demise was never suspected. Certainly her sons were stalwart men, of almost giant stature ; and if her later descendants are not all blessed with bounteous health, they are never heard to attribute their weakness to the sinful lacing practised by a female ancestor long before they were born.

Nor do these stays deserve to be blamed for present ills. While they are bad enough, they are better, and not worse, than the inventions that have succeeded them. The latter allow not an inch of empty space to be enclosed beneath their supple bones, and the many cunning gores fit themselves closely to every indentation and every curve ; while the former, by maintaining one unbroken slant in front from top to bottom, made the concave, hour-glass shape impossible, and allowed the stomach to preserve its proper contour. One can believe that there might have been comfortable breathing beneath them, even when they were brought well together by the leather string. Then, too, the old-fashioned stays were seldom worn till womanhood ; and the hardy life of a New England country girl in those early days had probably given the wearer of this garment that sturdy strength and vigor which enabled her to resist the evil influences of the dress of later life. And, after she became a matron, she put on her cuirass only occasionally, when she was to ride, perhaps, on her pillion, to the great town of Falmouth, six miles away, or to take tea with the doctor's wife, in the august presence of the parson. But now woman's form is not suffered to attain its natural size and strength; for corsets are put on in early girlhood, and worn steadily ever after, as a necessary part of the daily dress.

The corsets in use thirty or forty years ago, when the buckram stays had had their day, and before the products of French and German manufactories had become so common, were less objectionable than either of the other styles. Rows of soft wicking stitched into cotton jean took the place of the whalebones; and broad straps passing over the shoulders helped to support the weight of the clothing. In the front, the wooden busk still held its place.

This last feature of the old garment is usually

regarded as the worst article that woman ever invented for her own torment; but it had merits which should not be forgotten. Besides preventing a depression of the stomach from tight waist-bands, it was capable of being readily removed, when its wearer was at home and inclined to sit at ease; but the two iron bars, or clasps, which have taken its place, are too firmly fastened to the cloth to be withdrawn at will, and the discomfort they occasion must be endured without respite. In this connection, I think of Madame de Staël, sitting at table, as some one describes her, engaged in high and mighty discourse with her gentleman friends, — with Benjamin Constant, Schlegel, and perhaps Goethe himself,— and interrupting her disquisition on the philosophy of literature to crowd down an unmanageable wooden busk that would assert itself in spite of her efforts; till, discouraged at last, she drew it boldly forth and laid it on the waiter's tray to be removed. Even under that short bodice of hers, then, she thought it necessary to wear this instrument of torture. In matters of daily life and habit the wisest women appear to be little superior to their contemporaries.

Chemise. — I have shown why the corset must inevitably perish. The chemise is condemned for quite different reasons. No charge of compression or of inflexible shape can be brought against that: it errs in the other direction, if that can be said to err which appears to be wholly without use, and to offer no excuse for its existence. But its sins are not merely negative. It produces a great inequality in the temperature of the system, by affording no covering for neck and arms, while it furnishes loose folds of useless cloth to be wrapped about the body on its warmest part and under the tight dress-waist. There is an excess of material where it is not needed, over the lower portion of the trunk; and a deficiency where it is needed, over the extremities. The chemise can offer no support to any other garment; and in every respect a more absurd and worthless article of clothing could not possibly have been devised. Its rude and primitive construction should recommend it to no intelligence higher than that of South Sea Islanders, by whom it is doubtless worn. In civilized countries it is doomed to follow the corset to that limbo which dress-reformers will hereafter keep for the cumbrous and injurious habiliments of the past.

So much, then, we abandon: what do we retain, and of what will the reconstructed and hygienic attire consist? It is evident that no mercy can be shown to tight waists, built on the inverted pyramid plan; and that bindings for the waist must be utterly annihilated, if that shall prove possible; if it does not, they must be kept below the line of the waist, and terraced one above another.

Dividing our entire clothing into three divisions, — viz., underwear, skirts, external dress, — let us consider each in order.

The first division, the underwear, will in winter usually comprise two layers, — the flannel and the cotton garments; in summer, only one, — the cotton, or linen. Dealers in such goods tell us that the number of woollen under-garments sold to women in our country during the last ten years has been greatly in excess of previous sales; and it is gratifying to know that good sense in this department of dress is so rapidly on the increase. Many now wear such garments throughout the summer. We must, therefore, treat them as a part of the ordinary dress.

Flannel Underwear. — As commonly worn, this consists of two distinct garments, the drawers and the vest. The objections to their present arrangement are that one overlaps the other over half of the trunk of the body, while the only provision for the support of the lower is a binding pulling at the waist. Thus we have inequality of temperature and improper suspension of weight well provided for at the start.

The remedy for these evils is twofold. Retaining the two garments, we may shorten the upper till it only meets the lower; and may connect the lower directly with it at several points, so that the weight shall be borne by the shoulders, and not by the hips. Or we may have one garment woven entire, which shall take the place of the two commonly worn. This remedy is much to be preferred. And garments of this description are neither new nor strange. They have been manufactured for years in England, by the well-known firm of Cartwright & Warner, whose merino goods take the lead in every market. They are worn a great deal in Europe, and have been inported into this country at different times by nearly all the leading dry-goods houses of our principal cities, under the name of ladies' union flannel suits. Many American ladies have learned to like them during a stay abroad, and have since created some demand for them here; but in general they are little known. They are usually made of soft, thick merino wool; are high-necked and long-sleeved; and nothing more light, warm, comfortable, well-suspended and simple can be imagined. A representation of them will be found in the illustration which accompanies this Appendix, upon the card marked 4. Care must be taken in selecting these garments, if one wishes them to reach to the ankle under the stocking, as many only come well below the knee; while all those which have been found for sale in this country during the past season have had the objectionable feature of short sleeves. There is a long-sleeved variety, however, which is constructed throughout in strict accord with our four hygienic principles of dress; and this will, no doubt, be imported when the demand for it appears.

Those who have obliging friends travelling abroad can obtain these goods from shops in nearly all the leading cities of England and Scotland, and perhaps from the continent. Something similar can be formed by sewing together our ordinary knit under-vest and drawers just below the waist, and cutting off all superfluous cloth. Such a combination garment is a part of the hygienic suit worn by patients at the Health Home in Dansville, N. Y. Or a similar garment may be cut and made from unshrinking flannel cloth, and it will be found very comfortable.

Material. — No directions can be given concerning the quality and thickness of the flannel which shall comprise this suit : every lady will consult her own taste and habit; but, if the limbs be well covered, the material may be much thinner than is commonly worn. While our climate seems to require that we should protect ourselves well from its fitful changes, it is nevertheless true that many persons accustom themselves to more clothing than they really need. Rousseau held the opinion that men could dress in linen suits in winter, if they never enervated the system by wearing any thing more substantial; and though this notion, like many he cherished, was a little extravagant, there is no doubt that the less one wears the better, provided there is no sensation of cold. The thicker the clothing, the heavier it is to carry about, and the less readily does it permit the constant and invisible exhalations from the body to pass through its folds. Then a thin, light flannel cloth, such as the Scotch make, is often as warm as heavier goods. All flannel used for underwear should be light, warm, and porous; and in its manufacture a little cotton should be mixed with the wool, to prevent shrinking. Undergarments of very nice all-wool flannel, if washed every week, as of course they should be, soon become nearly impervious to air, and they ought then to be discarded. Those persons who object to flannel under-garments for summer may wear, instead, a suit of woollen gauze, or one of delicate knit silk. This last is the coolest and lightest of all materials; but it is not recommended to poor people, or to those who object to becoming such. Its durability, however, compensates in some measure for its high cost. For the first suit, almost any material should be preferred to cotton, as this has a peculiarly drying and heating effect upon the skin.

The union flannel suit just described is incomparably better than any other similar garment or garments, since it fulfils perfectly all the requirements of the four hygienic principles to be observed in dress. But, if two separable garments are preferred to one, we must provide for the joining of the two at several points somewhere below the waist, so that the weight of the whole may depend freely from the shoulders. The upper garment will be shortened till it extends only far enough to meet the lower, in order to avoid the inequality of temperature which the present adjustment of these garments necessitates.

Joining of Two Garments. — The more common and acceptable method of fastening the two garments together will be by buttons. Upon the straight lower edge of the vest, — when it has been made of the right length, and properly stayed either by a hem or a narrow facing, — sew four or six buttons; and in the top of the other garment make button-holes to correspond. The buttons should be of flat or concave surface, and about half an inch in diameter: one should be placed on each side of the vest; and between these, both on front and back, may be one or two others, set at equal distances apart. If the top of the lower garment is divided into two sections of equal length, there must be a horizontal button-hole in both ends of these sections; and the two button-holes on the same side will pass over the same button. The other button-holes will be vertical.

If the top, or binding, is of one piece, — as will be the case, if the garment is of the open pattern, — its two ends should meet at the front; and, if the vest also opens on the entire length of the front with a buttoned fold, a simple mode of lacing may be used to connect the two garments below the waist. In place of the buttons and button-holes, imagine common metal eyelet-holes to be set, an inch apart, in each garment. Lay the edge of the drawers upon the vest, with the eyelet-holes exactly corresponding in position. Then run a lacing or cord in and out, alternately, through the corresponding eyelet-holes, as may be seen in the illustration, card 9. There, however, the under row of eyelets is not set in the garment itself, but in a firm English tape an inch and a quarter broad, which is secured to the garment by two rows of stitching upon each edge, with the inner rows crossing at regular intervals. This gives a neater finish, and does not allow the cord to pass through to the under side, but it is at the expense of more labor. For the cord, any common corset-lacing will do, but a flat linen braid with a long metal at one end is best: to the other end, sew a loop of smaller braid: through this pass the lacing after it has gone through the first eyelet-holes, and draw it up closely; thus the end is secured. The other end, when the lacing is done, must be tied to a piece of tape sewed to the garment. The eyelets are very readily put in by a simple instrument made for the purpose, and in use in many stores and manufactories; or, in fine cloth, they may be punched by a stiletto and sewed over by hand, as in embroidery. This forms a smooth, pliable, and secure mode of fastening, connects two garments more closely than it is convenient to do with buttons, and thus distributes the weight and the pull equably over the shoulders. It renders the garments practically one while they are worn, and they might so remain; but it also allows that they may be made two, when it is desired to change either one and not the other.

The tops of all drawers and skirts should be without gathers or bindings. How these may be avoided in skirts will be hereafter shown. Superfluous cloth in the tops of drawers should be removed by gores : if properly cut, one gore on each side and two behind will suffice. Line the smooth top, thus made, with a facing sufficiently wide to hold button-holes or eyelets. Thus we rid ourselves of the work of putting on bindings, and of the clumsy, thick seam they give, while we lessen the cloth over the hips. In woollen material, however, two flat plaits of the cloth should be laid in place of two gores, somewhere on the sides or behind, as a provision against shrinkage.

White Cotton Suit. — The second layer of the underwear, made of cotton cloth, — or muslin, as it is called outside of New England, — usually comprises chemise and drawers. The chemise we abandon, and to the ordinary cotton drawers the same objections apply as to the flannel. The best substitute for both is a new garment called the chemiloon. It is represented on card 3 of the illustration, and is essentially the union flannel suit put into cotton. Like that garment, it covers the body with a uniform thickness; it is light and loose, with no gathers and no waist-band, and the whole weight hangs freely from the shoulders. It is very easily donned, may be either of the closed or open pattern, and can be adorned with all the embroidery and ornament that any one wishes to bestow upon it. It has been made and worn by many ladies, and they find it exceedingly comfortable. The material for it should be either common cotton cloth, linen, or Lonsdale cotton.

The only objection brought against the cotton chemiloon is its oneness; but this will prove, on wearing, to be the strongest point in its favor. For those who cherish the objection, however, a similar garment is provided, which is composed of two parts. Its upper section is a white basque waist, fitted well to the form, with a skirt five inches long; and it will be found represented on cards 5 and 6. It may be made of cambric for summer, of jean or twilled cotton for winter, or of common cotton cloth for all seasons. Buttoned upon this basque, below the waist-line, and just above the faced edge, are drawers, of the open style; and another tier of buttons above holds the underskirt, or the colored flannel drawers that sensible women wear in its place. A button higher still, on the middle of the back, serves in part to support the balmoral and to keep it in place. Instead of buttons, the mode of lacing already described may be used on this waist to advantage, for the lower garment at least. The inner faced edge of the basque serves to hold buttons for such attachments as stocking supporters. This arrangement of two separable garments probably furnishes the best possible substitute for chemiloons; but the superiority of the latter garment in simplicity of structure and of make, and in the facility and speed in dressing which it allows, is plainly apparent.

The stocking must be classed with this division of the apparel. It should be of warm woollen for winter, the warmer the better. The worsted balmoral stockings now so common are an improvement on the cotton hose in which it has been fashionable to shiver for the past few winters; but they are not as thick as they should be to ensure warm feet. For keeping the stocking in place, no garters are to be thought of. The highest order of English knighthood may adopt the garter as its badge, and may append to it the motto, *Honi soit qui mal y pense;* but no dress-reformer with a conscience can allow it a place in her wardrobe, and *not* to think evil of it is to be ignorant of the simplest truths that physiology teaches. Neither should the stocking be upheld by any elastic band that connects with a waist-band, for to compress the waist and to drag upon the hips is far worse than to compress the arteries below the knee. When a flannel suit is worn and is close-fitting at the ankle, the stocking may be drawn up over it, and secured at top by a button or small safety-pin. When the suit is loose at the ankle, the stocking will pass under it; and an elastic or tape band for its suspension must be attached to the upper portion of the garment at some comfortable point, so that the shoulders may serve for the support. For this purpose, a piece of stout tape, about a third of a yard long, may be folded over at the middle, so as to give the shape of a letter V with the included angle made acute. Upon the point of the V sew a button; sew the two upper ends of the V to the inside of the flannel or cotton chemiloon, just above the waist-line at the side; then the button will hang free from the garment, and will pull from the shoulder on both front and back. To the button on the lower point of the doubled tape attach some such stocking-supporter as will be seen depending from cards 3 and 4 in the illustration, or any other variety that may be found convenient. Some portion of this supporter should be elastic; and one end of the upright band should be doubled upon itself, by means of a movable slide or in some other way, so that it can be made longer or shorter according to the length of the stocking. The top of the stocking will be secured by buttons, or by a simple clamping contrivance upon the ends of the supporter.

Skirts. — This brings us to the second division of dress, — the skirts. They must be recognized as indispensable parts of our present attire ; but no one who makes a study of female gear can fail to see that they are essentially bad. Do what we will with them, they still add enormously to the weight of clothing, prevent cleanliness of attire about the ankles, overheat by their tops the lower portion of the body, impede locomotion, and invite accidents. In short, they are uncomfortable, unhealthy, unsafe, and unmanageable. Convinced of this fact by patient and almost fruitless endeavors to remove their objectionable qualities, the earnest dress-reformer is loath to believe that skirts hanging below the knee are not transitory features in woman's attire, as similar features have been in the dress of men, and surely destined to disappear with the tight hour-glass waists and other monstrosities of the present costume. Though our eyes may not be privileged to behold that promised land of the far future, wherein women shall move about, no longer swathed and hampered by floating raiment, but clothed simply and serviceably as men are clothed, we may yet express a conviction that any changes the wisest of us can to-day propose are only a mitigation of an evil which can never be done away till women emerge from this vast, swaying, undefined, and indefinable mass of drapery, into the shape which God gave to his human beings. It cannot be that we are to remain for all time the only creatures in the universe that destroy their natural appearance by artificial coverings. Animals, birds, and the whole brute creation add nothing to the apparel given them at birth; men, in all save a few countries, outline their forms by the dress they have chosen. Why, then, should woman, whose shape differs so little from that of her brother man, be expected to hide and confuse the contours of this common human form, as if they were a disgrace to her, and to her alone, and walk and work and live at perpetual disadvantage, because the wonderful mechanisms of the body, provided for her use in such work and such living, are clogged and weakened by masses of superimposed and useless drapery?

But since it is ordained that one half of European and American humanity may now appear in the shape which God gave them, — as bipeds, — and the other half may not, but must venture abroad only with a balloon-like expansion swinging loosely from the waist where it is tied, we cannot abolish skirts altogether from our present regenerated dress, as we do the corset, but must treat them as necessary evils. They seem intended for two purposes, — to keep the legs warm and to conceal them. As producers of warmth, they are utter failures: one half the cloth they require, if put into the form of drawers, will give twice the protection from cold, while the swinging motion of the skirts gives rise to a constant current of air beneath them. But nothing can take their place as inflating disfigurements. So let us be wise in our day and generation: let us seem to wear them, and yet wear only enough to save our appearance.

By skirts in this connection, I do not mean those of the outer dress, but all beneath them. Before speaking of their number, a few hints may be given in regard to lessening the weight of each. Put as little cloth into them as possible; make them no wider or longer than good looks require. The hem of the longest should be at least four inches from the ground, their tops two or three inches below the waist-line. From these tops, all superfluous material should be removed, by gores or other means, and not retained in gathers and plaits. Thus heat, as well as weight, will be diminished. Make them of the lightest serviceable cloth: the manufactured balmorals of felt are too heavy and too thick at the top, though admirably shaped. For white goods, cambric weighs much less than "muslin." If tucks must adorn them, let them be few and fine.

The number of these skirts will be one at least; for we are not providing for a gymnasium or bloomer suit, which requires none. This one will be a balmoral, or its substitute. The under-skirt would make a second, but it has given place to an extra pair of drawers, usually of colored material somewhat like the outer dress. Retaining the under-skirt and adding a hoop, we have three, — the largest allowable number.

When the under-skirt is dispensed with, the outer colored drawers which are worn instead should button upon the garment beneath, whether it be chemiloon or basque waist. Or they should form part of a second chemiloon of colored flannel, covering entirely the white flannel suit; and then the cotton chemiloon is omitted.

When the under-skirt is retained, it may be so constructed that there shall be no useless fulness at the top to be removed by gores. The cloth of which it is to be made should be cut semi-circular in shape, as outlined on card 7. A small piece of the same shape is cut from the centre, of sufficient size to leave the top of the desired width. Sew the two straight edges together, allowing for a placket, and the skirt is shaped completely, without other seams. The lower rounded edge cannot well be hemmed, and a facing would be troublesome to fit; therefore scallop the edge with the button-hole stitch, or set on a ruffle or a Hamburg edging with a narrow straight facing. Do not hem the selvages of the placket: they may be faced, if thought necessary, and a gusset set in for a stay. Face the top for button-holes, and hang the skirt upon the chemiloon beneath. The placket should be on the front, or on the left side near the front; and this is true of all skirts. They are then whole in the back; and a button-hole should be made directly behind, to meet a button set rather high on the seam of the waist, as represented in card 5. This button will prevent the skirt from twisting around or sagging down out of place, and it will also support half its weight. The cloth for the semicircular underskirt should be at least a yard wide: if only one is to be cut, two yards in length will be required; but, if there are to be two, three yards will be sufficient. When the skirt is to be of flannel that is liable to shrink, the top should be cut larger, to admit of a plait or two behind; and in that case the cloth must be wider than if the ordinary piece is removed from the centre.

When Prince Albert admired the red flannel skirt of the Scotch peasant girl, as she walked across the fields near Balmoral Castle, and his loving queen straightway ordered for herself a similar garment, she introduced a fashion which has resulted in a permanent gain to the dress of her sex. Colored woollen skirts became popular, and were soon manufactured ready for all to wear. In former times such skirts were of the quilted variety, made at home with much labor, gathered over the hips so as to contribute excessive heat to that region, and worn with weariness to the flesh. The plain tunnels of felt that have driven them out of existence are a great improvement on the straight quilted skirt; but they also are too heavy and too warm, and, moreover, they cannot usually be washed. It is better to substitute a skirt made of colored flannel, or other washable material, with its top made like the under-skirt just described, and with a straight, scant flounce set upon its lower edge, at the knee. If cloth is found sufficiently wide to cut the entire length of the skirt of this semicircular shape, the flounce will not be needed. Besides hanging from the button behind, the balmoral should be fastened to the front of the under-waist by two buttons; or it may be attached to suspenders.

Suspenders. — As to these articles, no style seems so good as the regular men's suspender of the Guyot pattern, stamped also as the *bretelles hygiéniques*. They cannot fall over the arms; and, however full the bust may be, they will, if properly adjusted, pass behind it. They are to be bought anywhere, as white, as delicate, as washable as one could wish. Ladies who have worn them for years pronounce them perfect. In the illustration, they are seen passing over cards 1 and 2. There are many new patterns of suspenders made especially for women, each claiming peculiar excellences. Dress-reformers have grown learned concerning them, but space fails us to rehearse their ins and their outs. We are firm in the faith that no one need be without a comfortable suspender of some sort, many women to the contrary notwithstanding. But it is always best to attach all the skirts to an under-waist, if that garment is able to carry them: if it is not, adopt suspenders for the balmoral.

The hoop seems banished from our attire; but it has survived many frowns of fashion since it monopolized the drawing-rooms of the reign of Queen Anne, and forced the courtly Addison to sneer at it in the Spectator; and it will no doubt return to us after a brief exile. Many persons will not abandon it even now, for, worn of diminished size, it brings advantages which compensate for its weight. It keeps the folds of the balmoral from clogging the lower limbs in walking, and it allows the tops of other skirts to be so attached to it as to prevent undue heating of pelvis and spine and to render all waist-bands unnecessary. This healthful and comfortable arrangement may be understood by a glance at card 8, and by a careful description. On the waist-binding of the hoop make the following changes: cut in it, directly behind, an upright button-hole, to match the button on the waist worn beneath it. On each side of the button-hole sew three buttons for holding common suspenders, placing the front ones just over the firm side terminations of the upper hoops. This will bring the front bands of the suspenders back under the arms, where they should be, for women. The loose end of the hoop-binding, which passes around the front to buckle on the left side, is now useless: cut it off. Thus your hoop will hang lightly from the shoulders and keep in place, with only half a binding. The suspenders, even, may be dispensed with, by buttoning the two ends of the remaining section of the binding upon the waist, at the sides. Now for the adjustment of under-skirt and balmoral. Make the plackets in both on the left side, near the front. The top of the semicircular under-skirt should be as large as the circumference of the upper hoops; in this faced top set eyelet-holes, about three inches apart; through these, lace the skirt upon the inside of one of the hoops near the top, and carry the lacing along on the front, to meet the other end of the lacing. These two ends of the lacing tie and untie. The balmoral is finished at the top with a semicircular binding or facing, which is to lie upon the hoops outside, quite near its waist-binding. It is held there in place by three buttons on the tapes of the hoop, one behind, and one on each side where the hoops end, with button-holes corresponding in the top of the skirt. The hoop is removed with the skirts upon it, when the balmoral is simply unbuttoned, and the under-skirt untied, on the side plackets. The lacing, when put in, is secured at each end by a knot tied over the last eyelet-hole. Thus one pair of suspenders and one button lift the whole skirts so lightly that the wearer is almost unconscious of their weight: they are nowhere felt at the waist, nor do they touch the body behind, below the waist, if the hoop projects, as it should, in something like a bustle, so as to make an air-chamber beneath the tops of the skirts.

This closes the catalogue of improved undergarments. Very many varieties might be mentioned, but these are the essential forms. Let me recapitulate, for the benefit of those who desire to wear the best assortment. Your first suit will be a chemiloon. In winter, it will be of flannel; in summer, of woollen gauze, silk, or cotton, but a chemiloon it will be. Above this, there may be another chemiloon of cotton, if the first suit is of a different material, and to this may be buttoned the under-skirt. But, if no under-skirt is worn, another chemiloon of colored flannel is added, or a pair of drawers made of colored woollen goods is buttoned to the chemiloon beneath. Then comes the balmoral hung upon the waist, upon suspenders, or upon a suspended hoop.

The Outer Dress. — The external costume forms the third and last division of the apparel.

For this no singular style is required, since our present fashions will supply a model which is the most healthful, convenient and artistic that is possible for us to-day: I mean the Gabrielle, or gored dress, with additions and modifications as represented in cards 1 and 2. It requires less cloth than any other, and is consequently lighter, as well as cheaper; its weight depends entirely from the shoulders; it has no band and no fulness at the waist; and its lines, flowing from shoulder to foot, blend bodice with skirt by graceful curves. This alone will form the house-dress. For the street superadd a polonaise, or, if you prefer, an over-skirt and a short sack. The color and material of these last garments may be different from the Gabrielle, which will appear to outward view only as the black under-skirt of the dress.

Would you make this costume? Buy a good paper pattern of the Gabrielle; cut off its train, rendering it as short as you can wear it, and still retain your peace of mind; trim some fulness from the gores behind and from the side-seams of the skirt; and fit its waist loosely to your form. Make it of black alpaca, cashmere, or silk, and it will be durable, and suited to all seasons. If you must yield to the tempter and trim the bottom, one broad flounce with a puffed heading should suffice; but let the trimming upon the neck, coat-sleeves and side-pockets be flat, so as to be well hidden beneath the polonaise. White cuffs, collar, and bright necktie will render it pretty for the house. Of cambric, with no waist-lining, it is that cool, light, washable robe of which we dream when the dog-days are upon us and Sirius rages. Let the polonaise be comfortably loose below the arms; hem the edge of its skirt; and, if the material be good, it will be sufficiently ornamented with handsome buttons upon the front, and a ruff, or what you will, about the neck. The over-skirt which is to be worn under the sack should have straps fastened to it and a loose binding, that it may not be felt at the waist.

Ornament. — The ornament used upon the dress should be light, durable, and simple. The heaviest trimmings known are kilt-plaits, and fringes of jet beads; and no approval of fashion should tempt one to wear them. The softness of lace, the gloss and swing of silken fringes, smooth, stitched bands of cloth or of braid, — these offer styles of adornment that are always tasteful and unobjectionable. There is no need of profuse trimmings where the material of the dress is rich and handsome; and, where it is cheap and simple, they are certainly out of place. Thomas Fuller says of the good wife, "She makes plain cloth to be velvet by her handsome wearing of it;" and a well-cut garment, of becoming shape and color, has in itself a beauty of contour and a play of fold which belong only to smooth and floating surfaces and lines. All ornaments worn upon the person should at least pretend to serve some useful purpose. There is no pretence of use in bracelets, ear-rings, necklaces, and such meaningless appendages, which are an inheritance from the barbarous tribes who hang rings in their noses as well as in their ears, smear their cheeks with red paint, wear strings of shells about their necks, and in all things mistake toggery for grace. Men have rid their dress of such unworthy gewgaws; and since we seem to follow slowly after their styles, adopting into our costume many minor features of their dress, we shall in time discard heathenish baubles for something less suited to childish tastes.

Waist of the Dress. — In the waist of the Gabrielle dress, biases should be recognized only so far as they are useful in outlining the natural form: they must never serve as accessories to that compression of the waist which has become so pernicious. Elizabeth Stuart Phelps, in that brilliant and suggestive monograph entitled "What to Wear," which has done such valiant service in the cause of dress-reform, does well to insist that plain biased waists have much to answer for in the tortures inflicted upon women by their dress. Her charges are none too strong. Nature is so directly at variance with this feature of our apparel, that it seems invented only to aid and abet the corset in its deadly work. We read in the old fairy story that, when Cinderella's haughty sisters would go to the prince's ball, more than a dozen laces were broken in endeavoring to give them a slender shape; and we know full well that without the biased waist their endeavors to make a presentable appearance would have been in vain. I have seen the Digger Indian women roaming the woods of California in a single garment, and that a calico dress with a biased waist. They could be indebted to civilization for but one article, and they chose that. But this feature of our attire has had its day. Before the growth of intelligence, it must inevitably disappear. The substitutes thus far provided have been straight waists girded with a belt drawn tight enough to keep the loose gathers down in place; so that one fault has been corrected by another equally bad. Belts for the outer dress are no more deserving of favor than those found in the under-wear. If any one cannot yet reconcile herself to the flowing curves of a loose Gabrielle waist, she may take refuge in an infinite variety of pretty little sacques, made beautiful with trimming; and with their adjunct of an overskirt, she can move as freely and breathe as deeply as she may wish.

Length of Skirt. — The length of the skirt can even now be very much shortened, without attracting attention or bringing annoyance to the wearer. When the bloomer dress was devised, high boots for women were not known; and for the long gap between skirt and boot a visible pantalette of the Turkish pattern was provided. This made a conspicuous feature of the short dress. But, if a dress-skirt reaches the tops of our present boots, it is a long way from the ground. A skirt of that length will look graceful and becoming to all sensible observers. But, were it necessary to make a choice between cleanliness and grace, no lady should fail to choose the former, especially when health and comfort accompany it. Many persons pause to look after any display of the latest styles, any fresh, beruffled train sweeping the sidewalk; and the wearer appears in no wise dismayed or saddened by the attention she excites. Cannot we show as much heroism in the cause of good sense as she shows in the cause of folly, and endure an occasional glance at the novelty of a short, trim skirt and unencumbered feet? Fashion finds plenty of followers to do her bidding: why cannot reformers equal them in fortitude and composure?

Wraps. — For outer garments, the short sacque is the most serviceable. The shawl has antiquity and grace to recommend it: we remember how universally its shape entered into the component parts of the female dress of the Greeks, in what rich folds of drapery it sweeps down from the shoulders, and how, in the hands of a Lady Hamilton, it may lend a charm even to the swaying motion of the dance that bears its name; but it impedes the movement of the body in walking, covers the arms till they are nearly useless, and crowds about the neck. When we have a mind to be statuesque at all hazards, or when we can rest at ease on carriage cushions, or take a siesta at home, it may be made available; but, when we wish to walk or to work, it can be nothing but an encumbrance. Then a simple, sleeved garment is far preferable.

Clothing of the Extremities. — The hands in winter should never be confined in a muff; nor should furs be worn about the neck. Mittens are better than gloves for warmth; and women should learn to move their arms freely at the side, instead of keeping them bent, with the hands pinioned at the waist. The sleeve has reached perfection in the close coat-sleeve, cut high on the shoulder, so as to give freedom of movement to the shoulder-joint. We are indebted to the French for so many pernicious fashions, that we may thank them for a style as sensible as this.

I need not say that a low-heeled, broad-soled boot or shoe, of soft, stout leather, not too loose or too tight, is requisite to the proper clothing of the foot, and to an easy and elastic gait. There may be a variety in the shoes to be worn on different occasions; and they should be changed often, as should also the stocking, owing to the moisture of the foot. We may not have as large an array of shoes as the historian Prescott kept for his own use; but slippers for the house, made of thick cloth for winter, "Newport ties," and boots of several varieties of make, seem essential to daily comfort. Calf-skin is the best leather for ordinary wear; but, while goat-skin is no protection against wet, its porous nature allows the exhalations from the foot to pass off freely. Nothing should be suffered to interfere with this function of the skin. Cork-soles covered on one surface with enameled cloth, and rubber shoes, are too impervious to the air. Indeed, rubber shoes, and especially rubber boots, should very seldom be worn. The Maine lumbermen secured rubber boots for themselves as soon as these articles appeared in the market, thinking thus to keep their feet dry while rafting logs on the Penobscot; but they soon found their feet more damp than before, and were obliged to abandon the boots.

The exhaled moisture of the foot, instead of passing off into the air, was again absorbed, to the injury of the system. In a January thaw, or on a glare of ice, rubbers are indispensable; but they should be removed as soon as possible.

For the head, a soft, light hat seems perfection; and one may not deny it the ornament of a curling ostrich feather; though if birds would only teach us the art of keeping their plumes in curl in damp weather, so that we could wear them confidently in a fog, there would be no drawback to their grace and beauty. That conglomeration of bows, muslin flowers, buckles, feathers, lace, and beads, usually heaped upon the useless articles called hats, presents a style of composite architecture not edifying to behold. It is less beautiful and becoming than the plain hat which men wear; but the latter might borrow to advantage a few of our useless feathers. The width of the hat-brim should render parasol and veil unnecessary; but it should not be wide enough to become unmanageable in the wind.

When women can lay aside all the braided tresses that belong to another, as well as part of their own, and can show a well-shaped head in short, curling locks with their graceful curves and rings, they will have added inexpressibly to their comfort, health, and good looks.

Such is the apparel which intelligent care would proffer to the women of our time. Clothe yourselves thus, and life is no longer a burden. You look like other women, and no one suspects that you are not as miserable as they; but you breathe where they gasp, the library books on the top shelf are within your reach, and when a friend asks you to walk a mile you are ready to go with him twain.

Even in this day of pinching corsets and entangling trains, women are fast learning to respect the nature in themselves; and they will, ere long, forswear bands and burdensome toggery, and roam the meadows and walk the streets, if not kirtled like Diana and her nymphs when equipped for the chase, yet with a dress too simple to absorb their minds, too easy to cripple their movements, too healthful to rob their cheeks of a bloom which should be as fresh and rosy as that of the clover-tops they tread.

A.

Abdomen, contents of	102
effect of heat on	11, 13, 127
pressure on	16, 79, 110, 111
American women, dress of	7, 38, 97, 124, 135
Anatomy of body	100
Antagonism between health and custom	125
Appendix	xviii
Art education	167
Associated effort	4, 96
Association on dress	vi, 2
Austrian laborers, dress of	15

B.

Bands at waist	13, 14, 17, 39, 61, 112, 113, 115, 127, 216
Beauty in dress	37, 79, 82, 140, 141, 155, 162, 168
nature	79, 148
Bloomer dress	viii
Body, anatomy of	110
cavities of	46, 61, 62, 101
effect of cold on	10, 12, 85, 117
flexibility of	206
lack of respect for	130, 139
mechanisms of	92, 99, 138
physiology of	100
structure of	43, 100, 101, 204

INDEX OF TOPICS.

Body, temperature of 10, 71, 83, 114, 116
    vertical bearing of 76, 110
Blood, circulation of . . . 50, 52, 58, 72, 76, 104, 106
Boots 39, 63, 73, 75, 116, 249
Busk 213

C.

Cavities of body 46, 61, 62, 101
Chemiloon 225
Chemise 215
Children, dress of 26, 83
Circulation of blood . . . 50, 52, 58, 72, 76, 104, 106
Circulatory system 102
Coeducation 21
Cold on body, effect of 10, 12, 85, 117
Congestion of organs 10, 53, 59, 71, 117, 118
Converts to truth 5, 123
Corsets, as furnishing support 49, 200
    how improved 114, 207
    as preventing respiration 54, 56
        pressure from bands 16, 17, 109, 202
    steel bars in front of 20, 23, 110, 206
    as worn tight 57, 59, 77, 112, 164, 193, 203, 205, 208
        by children 55
Costume, external . . . . vii, 3, 44, 119, 187
Cotton suit 225
Custom antagonistic to health 125

D.

Diaphragm 51, 56, 108, 115
Digestive system 102

Diseases of women 21, 25, 58, 62, 79, 129, 130
Dress of American women 7, 37, 97, 124, 135
    artistic element in 147, 154, 166
    of Austrian laborers 15
    beauty of 37, 82, 148
    of children 26, 83
        Christian nations 130
    conventional 136
    of men and women contrasted 149, 153
    deference paid to 9, 65
    dissatisfaction with 1
    of earnest women 31, 33, 37, 136
        Eastern nations 131, 133
    employment furnished by 27, 92
    evils of present . . 13, 43, 68, 70, 74, 82, 95, 177
    extravagance in 8, 89, 93
    external 3, 44, 64, 119, 187
    of First Empire 143
    Greek and Roman 130, 142, 201
    should be healthful 138
    for holiday occasions 30, 149, 158
    as impeding motion 72, 75, 78
    improvements in 39, 60, 77, 114, 119, 162, 164, 168
    of infants 83
    as lacking beauty 139, 145
    material of 27, 34, 40, 71, 219
    of men 37, 64, 72, 148, 154, 162
    as affecting mind 70, 90, 94
            morals 8, 64, 66, 92, 94
    of mothers 18, 119, 131
    permanent styles in 33
    physician's duty concerning 85
    picturesque element in 147, 158
    primal use of 71

Dress of the rich 6, 8, 66, 88, 91
    reform in, need of . 6, 44, 68, 70, 82, 88, 98, 120,
    128, 135, 145
    worn in Sandwich Islands 131, 143
    in sick-room 40
    simplicity in 163
    specialists in 34
    subordination of 41
    tight 49, 52, 57, 80, 126
    unequal thickness of 11, 12, 127
    uniformity in 44, 64
    for walking 70, 80, 164
    weight of 25, 63, 78, 130
    of Western nations 133
        working women 7, 136, 157

E.

Earnest women, dress of 31, 33, 37
Economy in dress 172
Education of girls, physical 22, 120
Employment furnished by dress 27, 92
Evils of present dress 13, 43, 68, 70, 74, 82, 95
External costume 3, 44, 64, 119, 187, 241
Extravagance in dress 8, 89, 93
Extremities, clothing of 249

F.

Fashion, fickleness of . . . . xii, 165
    foreign . . . . xii, 97
    improvements in 162, 164, 168
    tyranny of 23, 42, 78, 135
Feet, clothing of 39, 63, 73, 75, 84, 116, 191

Flannel underwear 114, 217
Flexibility of ribs 48, 102
Functions in health 100, 103, 116, 121

G.

Garments, number of 3, 28
         ready made 168
Garters 76, 113, 228
Girls, physical education of 22, 120, 174, 176

H.

Habit, effect of, on system 57, 81, 112
Hair, dressing of 24, 40, 252
Health of women 75, 77, 98, 129, 132
Heels high 75, 165
Hips, weight on 14, 17, 39, 61, 62, 197
Holiday dress 30, 158
Hoops 238
Hygienic dress, need of 6, 45, 120

I.

Ill-health of women . . 43, 68, 75, 77, 98, 129, 132, 135
Improved undergarments 39, 60, 77, 114, 119
Infants, dress of 83

J.

Joining of two garments 222

K.

Kidney 12, 63

L.

Laborer, elevation of the 27, 91
Lectures on dress . . . . v, xv
Leggins 39, 116
Limbs, proper clothing of . . 12, 116, 118, 127, 146, 191
Liver 51, 77
    effect of pressure on 16
Looseness at waist 80, 83, 193
Lungs 49, 106, 108
    effect of pressure on 57, 109

M.

Material of dress 14, 27, 34, 40, 71, 219
Men, dress of, improvement in 162
    its lack of beauty . . . . . . 148, *sq.*
    its material 37
    as serviceable 64, 72, 148
    unfriendly to dress-reform 9, 170
Mental growth of women . . 1, 38, 64, 69, 87, 133, 136
Mind, effect of dress on 70, 90, 94
Missions of men and women 156
Morals, effect of present dress on . . 8, 64, 66, 92, 94
Mothers, effect of present dress on 18, 119, 128, 123, 131
Motion impeded by dress 72, 75, 78

N.

Nature, beauty in 79, 148
Need of dress-reform . . 6, 45, 68, 70, 82, 88, 98, 120
Nervous centres 19, 101, 110, 128
Number of garments worn 28

O.

Opholzer, Professor, anecdote of	32
Ornament	243
Outer dress	3, 44, 64, 119, 187

P.

Panier	63, 79
Pelvic region	196
Permanent styles of dress	33
Physical education of girls	22, 120
laws, unvarying	121, 128
Physicians, duty of concerning dress	34, 85
Physiology	100
Poor helped by sewing	27, 92
Pressure on limbs	76, 113
liver	16
lungs	57, 109
ribs	16, 47, 108
stomach	19, 110
womb	16
Principles, hygienic	190

R.

Reform in dress, need of	6, 45, 68, 70, 82, 88, 98, 120, 125, 128, 135, 145
how effected	44, 86, 96, 121, 122, 166, 173
Respiration	103, 107, 115
effect of, on blood	52, 107, 108
Ribs, effect of pressure on	16, 47, 108, 143
flexibility of	45, 48, 54, 102
Rich women, dress of	8, 66, 88, 91

S.

Sewing, effect of	27, 90, 94
Shoes	39, 63, 73, 75, 115
Shoulders, support from	39, 44, 55, 61, 63, 73, 81, 114, 115, 126, 193, 197
Skating	22
Skin, function of	11, 40, 119
Skirts, for infants	84
length of	15, 44, 63, 78, 79, 84, 115, 144, 163, 247
long, uncleanliness of	79, 165
of peasant costumes	37
trailing	35, 38, 80, 142
weight of	11, 17, 21, 63, 78, 196, 230
Solar plexus	19, 110
Specialists in dress	34
Stays, old-fashioned	210
Stockings	39, 115, 227
Stomach, effect of pressure on	19, 110
Structure of body	43, 101
Subordination of dress	32, 41, 88
Suspenders	14, 115, 237
Systems, circulatory	102
digestive	102
excretory	103, 119
respiratory	103, 107, 115

T.

Temperature of body	10, 71, 83, 114, 116, 127, 191, 195
Tight dressing	49, 52, 57, 80
Time given to dress	28, 70, 86
Trailing skirts	10, 35, 38, 80, 160
Tyranny of fashion	23, 42

U.

Undergarments, importance of . . . . xiv, 119, 188
                improved 3, 38, 60, 77, 114, 119, 188, 216
Uniform styles of dress 44, 64, 179, 189
         temperature of body 191, 194
Uterine diseases, increase in 14, 111, 118
Uterus 16, 18, 76

V.

Veils 4
Vertical bearing of body 76, 110

W.

Walking 75, 78, 115, 146
Walking-dresses 79, 80, 164
Waist, bands around 17, 61, 80, 112, 115
      cotton 226
      looseness at 80, 81, 83, 193, 245
      standard size of 144
Weight of dress 25, 63, 78, 192
      on hips 14, 39, 61, 62
Women, diseases of 21, 25, 58, 62, 79
      ill-health of 75, 77, 98, 129, 132
      mental growth of . 1, 38, 64, 69, 87, 133, 136
      not naturally weak 21, 129
Work honorable for women 30, 93
Working women, dress of 7
         dress of Austrian 15
Wraps 248

NOTICE.

THE Committee on Dress-Reform have extended their work by opening in Boston an accessible and attractive room, which is intended to serve for a bureau of information on all matters connected with dress-reform. They have provided it with an intelligent and earnest attendant, put into it specimens of nearly every article of under or outer wear which they have examined and approved, are now ready to exhibit these to all who may come to see, to manufacture them for all who may wish to buy, and to furnish patterns, instructions, or any aid that may be sought. They purpose to render this room a convenient centre and exchange for all dress-reformers who may have ideas or inventions to contribute to the cause, or who may wish to take away those of others. This room will be found at 25 Winter Street, over Chandler's dry-goods store, room 15.

It is intended that the room shall be self-supporting; but, as this is a benevolent enterprise, only such profit will be asked on the articles sold as shall be necessary to ensure the payment of running expenses. The labors of the committee will of course be gratuitous; and they will keep all expenses at a low figure, in order that the garments which they seek to introduce may be put within reach of all. To this end, also, they will be willing to provide the plainest and cheapest material, as well as the richest.

The full suit of these garments will comprise the entire flannel under-suit of new and improved pattern, manufactured in this country, according to designs furnished by the Committee; chemiloons of all varieties of make, in muslin, cambric, and flannel; basque under-waists, with other garments properly attached; suspenders of all sorts; hoops with other skirts affixed so as to avoid waist-bindings, under-skirts, balmorals, Gabrielle dresses, and whatever else goes to the making up of a well-dressed woman, according to the light of the new dispensation. Nothing will be furnished which the Committee do not consider to be constructed, in all essential particulars, on strict hygienic principles. They will never forget that they are missionaries and not merchants; but they will spare no pains to render the garments they furnish acceptable, and therefore beneficial.

Orders sent must give explicit directions as to style, material, size, and ornament, in order to prevent the delay resulting from explanatory correspondence. They should be addressed to Dress-Committee, 25 Winter Street, Boston, Room 15; and a stamp should be enclosed, if reply is called for. Articles ordered will be forwarded by express at the expense and risk of persons ordering them.

Hitherto it has been, Dress-reform made possible; hereafter it shall be, Dress-reform made easy. That, surely, will be a great gain.

For the Committee.

Messrs. Roberts Brothers' Publications.

WOMAN IN AMERICAN SOCIETY.

BY ABBA GOOLD WOOLSON.

Price $1.50.

Extract from a letter by Wm. Lloyd Garrison.

I am so pleased with what you have written, not only as a specimen of admirable English composition, but for its rare good sense, its excellent and much needed advice, its delicate satire, its clear perception of what belongs to true womanhood, and its vigorous treatment of the various topics described from "The School Girl" to "The Queen of Home," that I cannot withhold an expression of my respect for your talents and high appreciation of the service you have rendered your sex.

Extract from a letter from Geo. S. Hillard.

I think them excellent, combining sound sense with feminine delicacy of observation.

G. B. E. in Boston Transcript.

Here is a powerful plea for a higher and more complete education for women; for an education which shall develop her powers of mind and of body, more justly and more thoroughly, and fit her for taking in society the high position for which God has created her. This book ought to be in the hands of every girl who desires to live a healthy, happy life, and of every mother who would have her daughter prepared for such a life.

From the Christian Register.

This is a thoroughly good book, — good in style, good in thought, good in its practical purpose, its shrewd sense, its exquisite humor, its delicate sarcasm, its honesty, and its earnestness. Every one of its twenty essays touches some social failing and hints some useful improvement.

The criticism, sharp and frank as it is, is never malicious or cynical. There is no pedantry, though the author is evidently expert in lore both ancient and modern; no sickly sentiment, and, what is rare in a lady's book, no poetical quotation.

The longest chapter in the book, and, as a piece of description, the finest, is the nineteenth, on "Grandmothers' Houses." This is painting from the life, and with a minuteness and finish worthy of the most accomplished of the Dutch or Flemish masters. Whittier's "Snow-Bound" is not more complete in its kind.

From the Boston Globe.

It consists of twenty short, sensible, witty, and vigorous essays, directed chiefly against the follies of the sex.

From the Boston Journal.

She writes so keenly at times as to suggest comparison with the author of the "Saturday Review" papers on woman; with this marked difference, that, while the criticisms of the latter are bitter and unsparing, those of Mrs. Woolson, however sincere, evince always the generous purpose which underlies them, and show the author's appreciation of woman's real worth and the opportunities within her reach.

From the Boston Saturday Evening Gazette.

There is that in it that needed to be said, and had not been said before, in any writing that had come under our observation, so well as she has expressed it here.

Sold everywhere. Mailed, postpaid, by the Publishers,

ROBERTS BROTHERS, BOSTON.

Messrs. Roberts Brothers' *Publications.*

THORVALDSEN:
HIS LIFE AND WORKS.

By EUGENE PLON.

Translated from the French by I. M. LUYSTER. Illustrated by Two Heliotypes from Steel Engravings by F. GAILLARD, and Thirty-five of the Master's Compositions, drawn by F. GAILLARD, and engraved on wood by CARBONNEAU. Second American Edition. One handsome square 8vo volume, cloth, gilt and black-lettered, gilt top, bevelled boards. Price $4.00.

From the Boston Daily Advertiser.

M. Eugene Plon has written a complete and fascinating biography of Thorvaldsen. This great Danish sculptor adopted Winckelmann's theories of art, and endeavored so faithfully to put them into practice that his sculpture is the best and truest expression of them ever given. M. Plon gives a clear and singularly interesting sketch of the progress of the fine arts in Denmark, and the influence of the French school there; and he awakens in the reader a genuine interest in the principles of art which guided Thorvaldsen in the method of his work, and in its extraordinary success. The translation now published by Roberts Brothers is made by Miss Luyster from a revised copy, given by the author, and is in every way admirable. The illustrations were printed in Paris expressly for this translation: they are on India paper, from the original blocks, and are clear and delicate. The frontispiece is from Horace Vernet's portrait of Thorvaldsen. The two masters were warm friends, and charming things are told of their appreciation of and admiration for each other.

From the Golden Age.

Thorvaldsen's Life belongs to romance, but his genius is an inspiration of art. The story of the man is pathetic as well can be: the history of the artist is full of heroism, aspiration, and triumph. Thorvaldsen's biography is a hard one to write delicately; indeed, it is hard to write at all, because a true biography must come out of sympathy and admiration, and there is much in his conduct that it is impossible to extenuate, and difficult to tell in a way that shall not offend the modern reader. M. Plon has done his work well. He has told the story unexceptionably, and interpreted the acts of the master from the spirit, the genius, the destiny of the man rather than by conventional rules. He is an admirable interpreter of the great Northman's artistic spirit and achievements. The volume, with its finely executed cuts and complete account of the great master's works, is a real contribution to the literature of art, and well calculated to foster the growing interest in art studies and pursuits.

Sold everywhere. Mailed, postpaid, by the Publishers,

ROBERTS BROTHERS, BOSTON.

www.ingramcontent.com/pod-product-compliance
Lightning Source LLC
Chambersburg PA
CBHW032055220426
43664CB00008B/1002